Grandmaster Ted Gambordella

The 100 Best
Stretch Tube Exercises

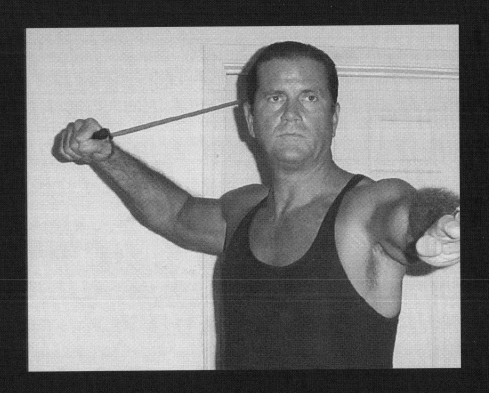

 The Ultimate Martial Arts

Shoulder Exercises

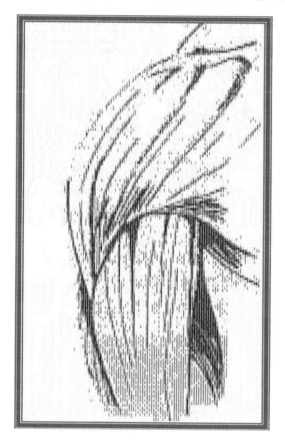

Do all exercises 6 to 8 times. 3 to 4 sets.

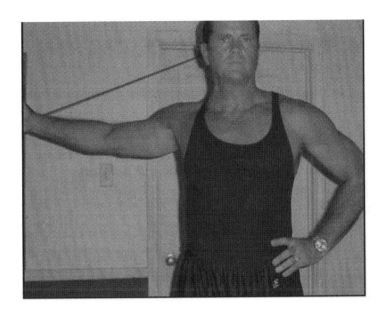

We start with the tube held high and extend our arm out to the side, then pull it down and forward to work the upper shoulders and chest.

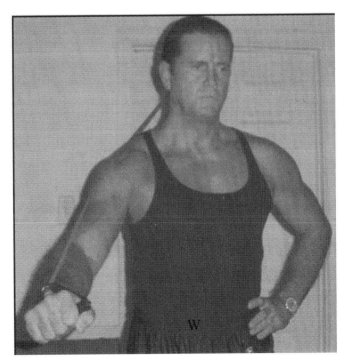

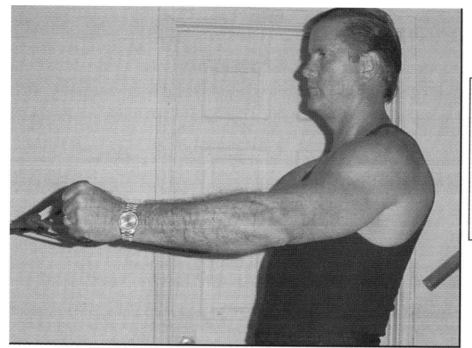

Here we have both arms extended at shoulder height in front of the body and then we pull them directly apart to the sides

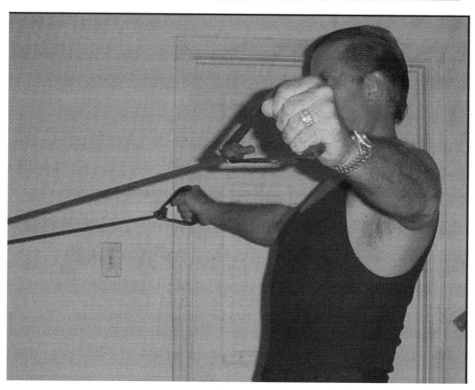

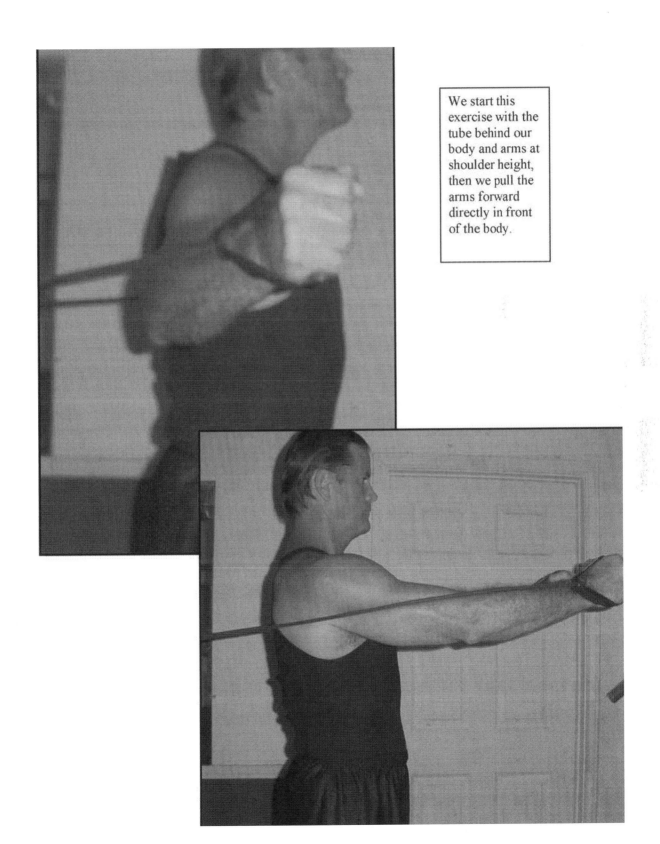

We start this exercise with the tube behind our body and arms at shoulder height, then we pull the arms forward directly in front of the body.

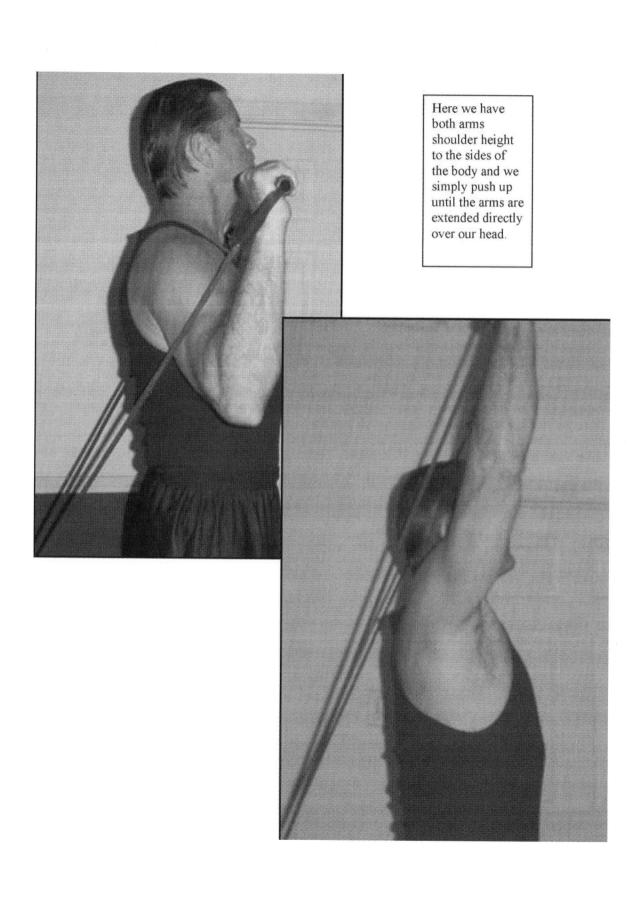

Here we have both arms shoulder height to the sides of the body and we simply push up until the arms are extended directly over our head.

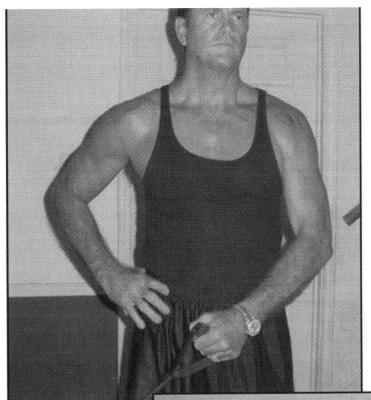

Here we have both we have arm in front of the body with the tube to the side. We then extend the arm across our body and out directly to the side.

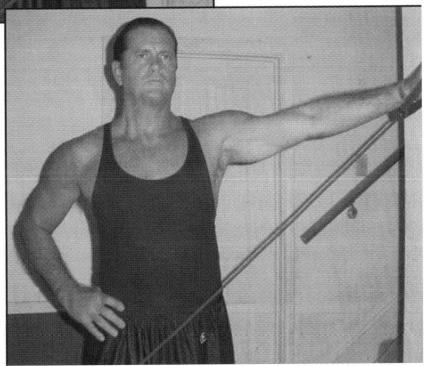

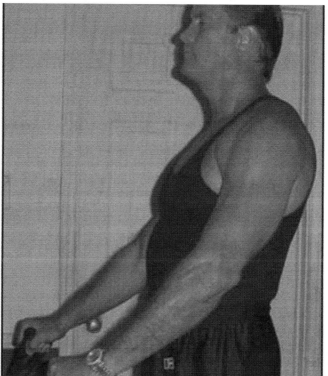

Here we have both arms down in front of the body, we then pull each arm up and to the side, alternating arms for one set.

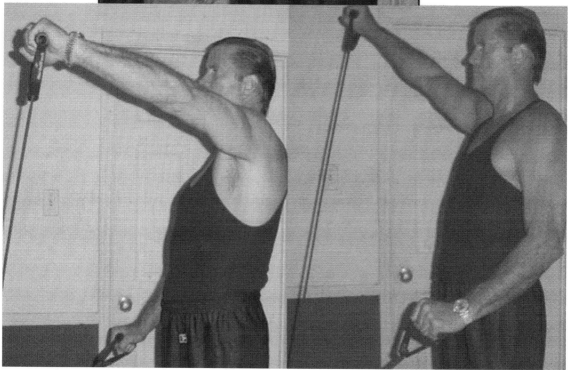

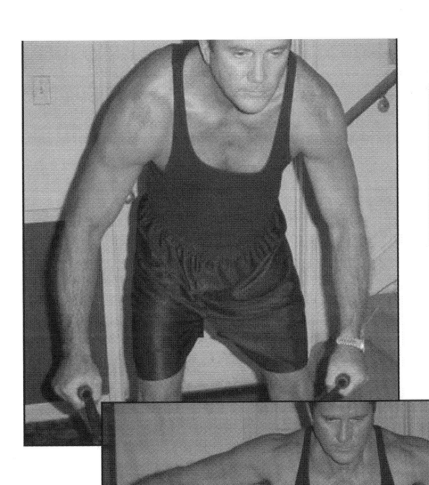

Here we have both arms extended down in front of the body and we are slightly bent over, then we pull back the arms and directly to the sides.

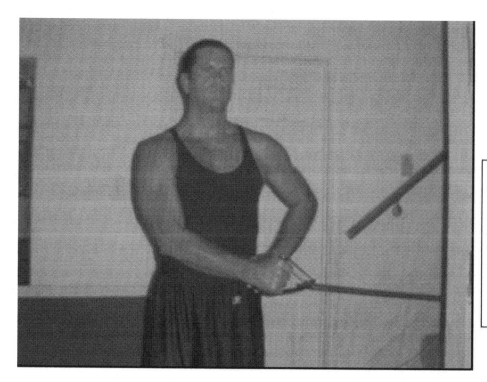

Here we the arm extended down and in front of the body, then we pull the arm up and to the side,.

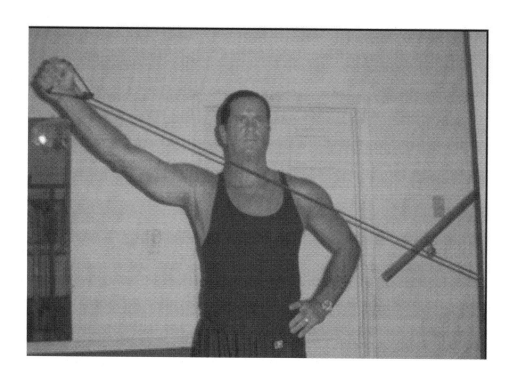

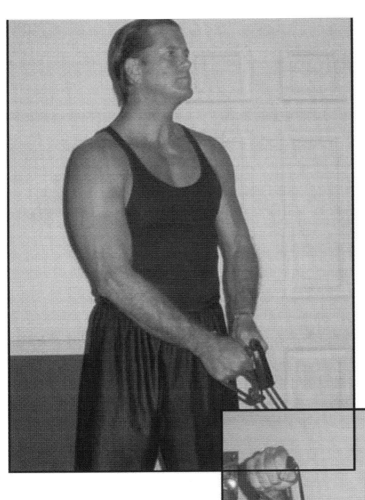

This is a variation of the previous move, but now both arms are down in front of the body and then we separate the arms one going up and the other going back.

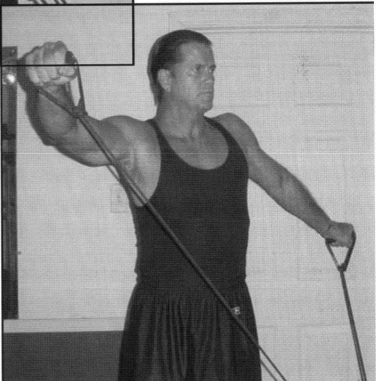

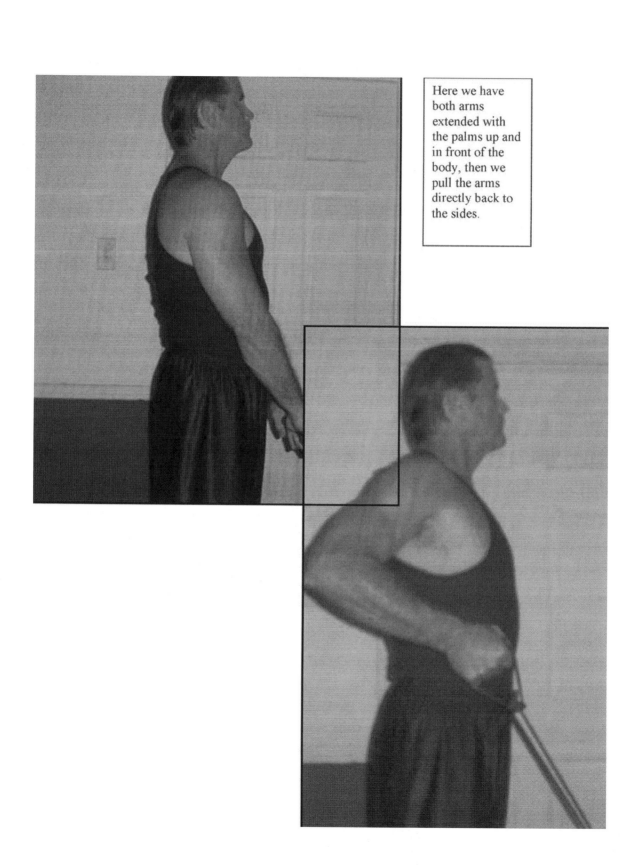

Here we have both arms extended with the palms up and in front of the body, then we pull the arms directly back to the sides.

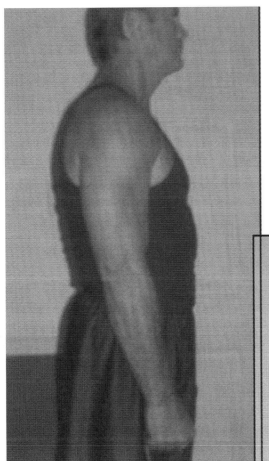

Here we have both arms extended down to the sides of the body and then we lift our shoulders up and roll the in small circles.

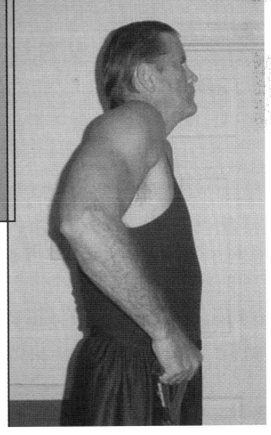

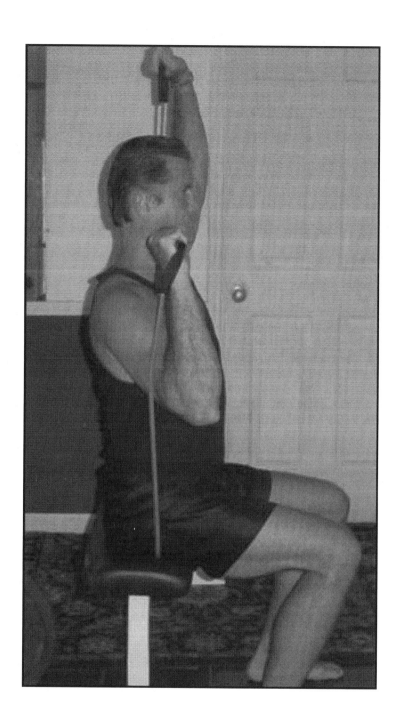

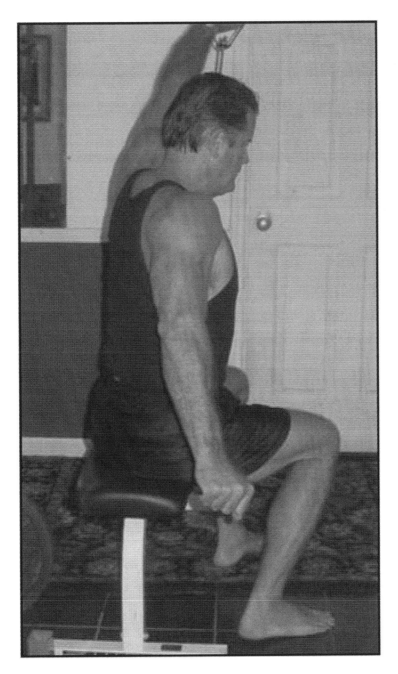

Here we are sitting and we extended one arm up and to the side and one arm back.

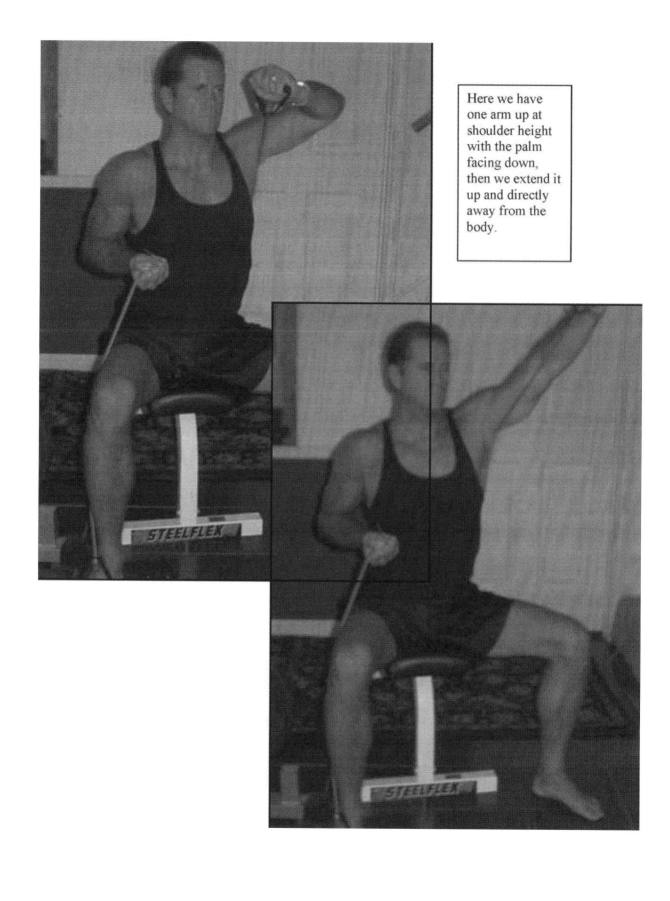

Here we have one arm up at shoulder height with the palm facing down, then we extend it up and directly away from the body.

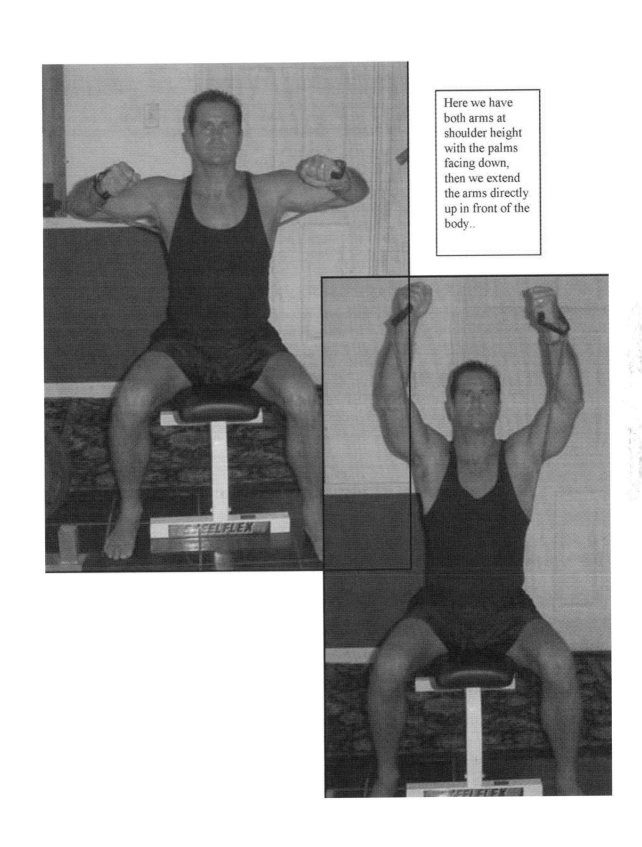

Here we have both arms at shoulder height with the palms facing down, then we extend the arms directly up in front of the body..

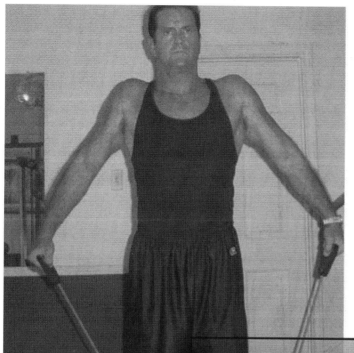

Here we have both arms extended down to the side of the body with the palms facing out, then we pulls the arms up directly in front of the body.

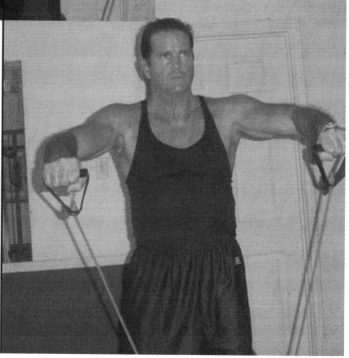

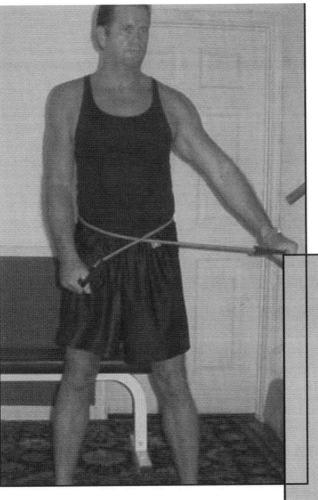

Here we have one arm out to the side and one arm holding tight to the waist. Then we pull the arm up and in front of the body. Notice how I have crossed the tube around my body to hold it secure for the exercise.

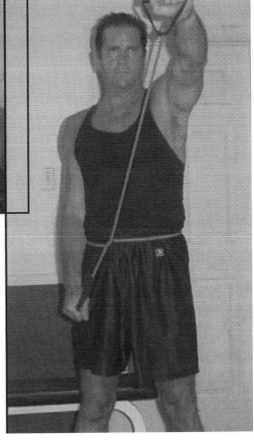

Here is the same exercise done with both arms. We extend the arm sback and directly away from the body..

Notice how I have crossed the tube around my body to hold it secure for the exercise.

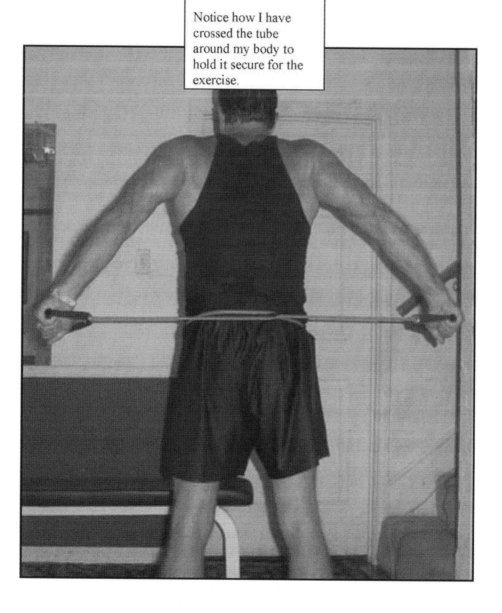

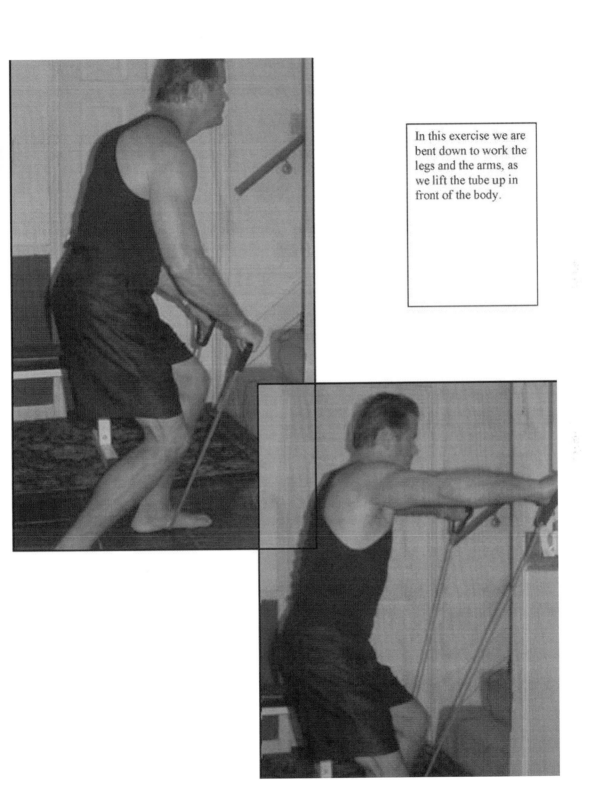

In this exercise we are bent down to work the legs and the arms, as we lift the tube up in front of the body.

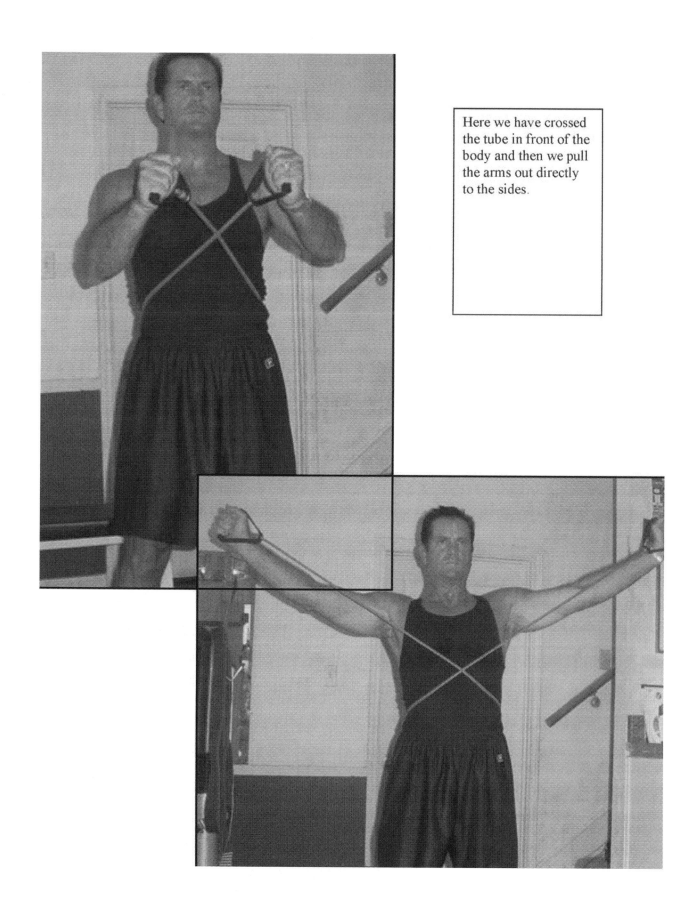

Here we have crossed the tube in front of the body and then we pull the arms out directly to the sides.

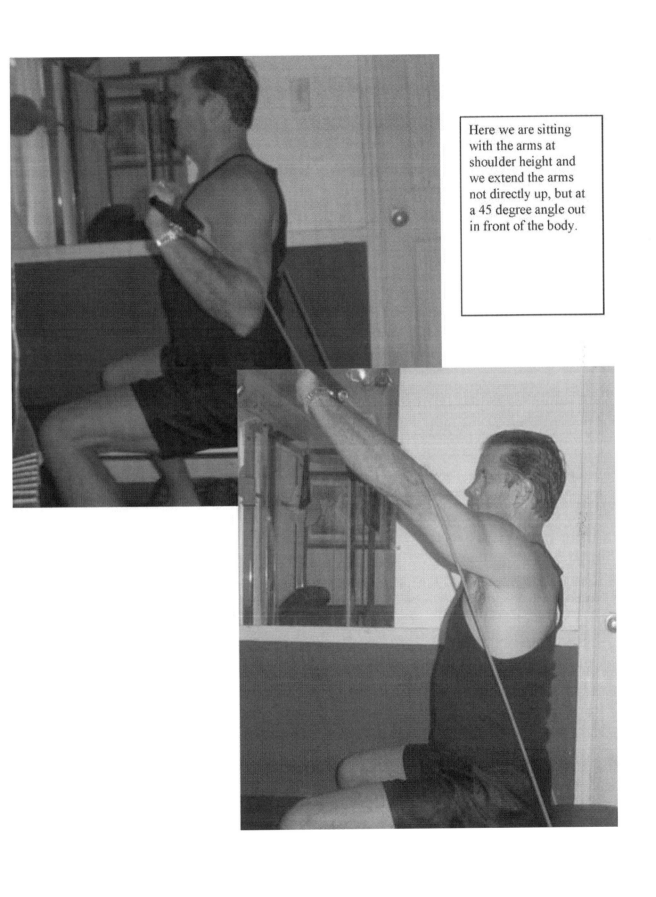

Here we are sitting with the arms at shoulder height and we extend the arms not directly up, but at a 45 degree angle out in front of the body.

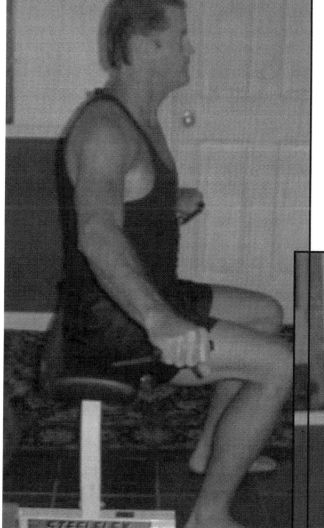

Here we are sitting with the arms already out to the sides and then we extend the arms up all the way up and to the side.

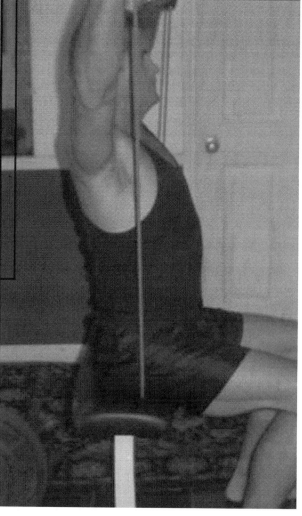

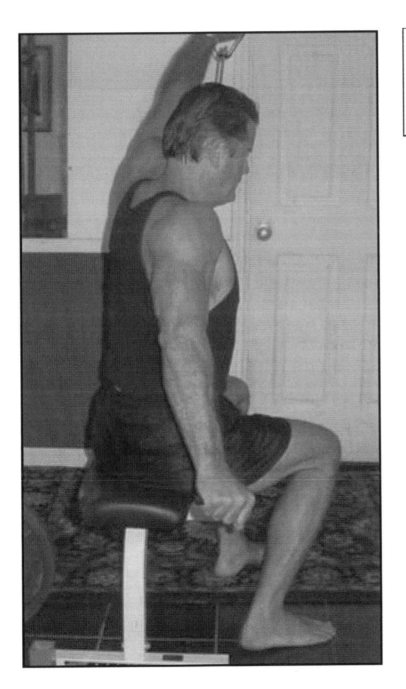

This is a variation with one arm going up and one arm going back. .

Here are lying down with the leg holding the tube and the arms up, then we pull the arms back across the body fully to the sides.

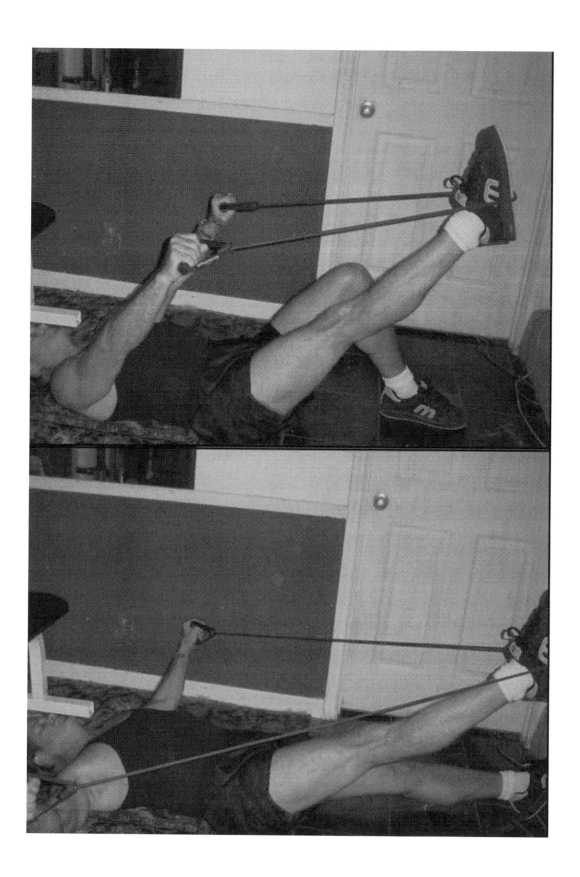

Abdominal Exercises

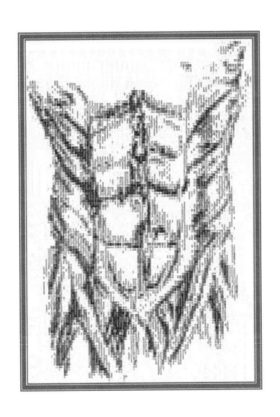

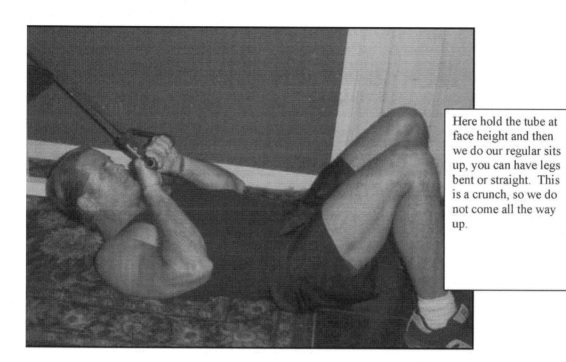

Here hold the tube at face height and then we do our regular sits up, you can have legs bent or straight. This is a crunch, so we do not come all the way up.

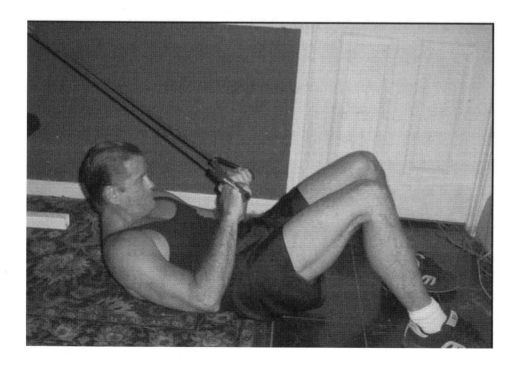

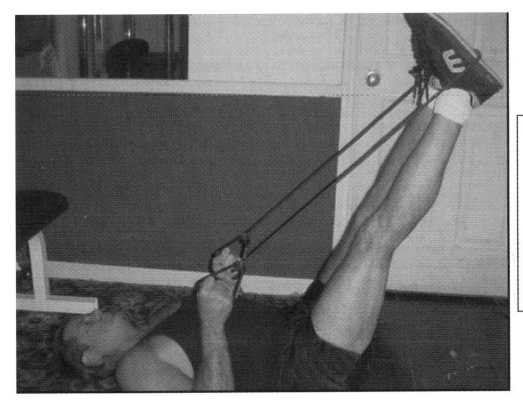

Here we work the lower abs by holding the legs up wit the tube and then extending them down to the ground.

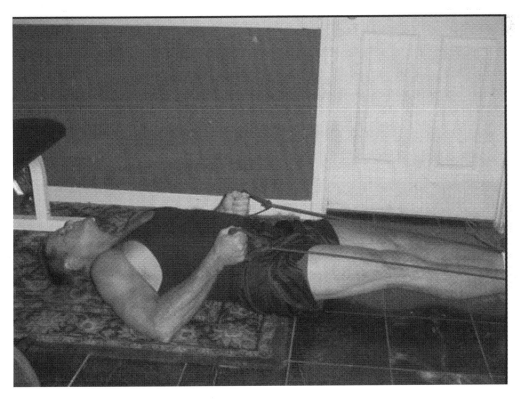

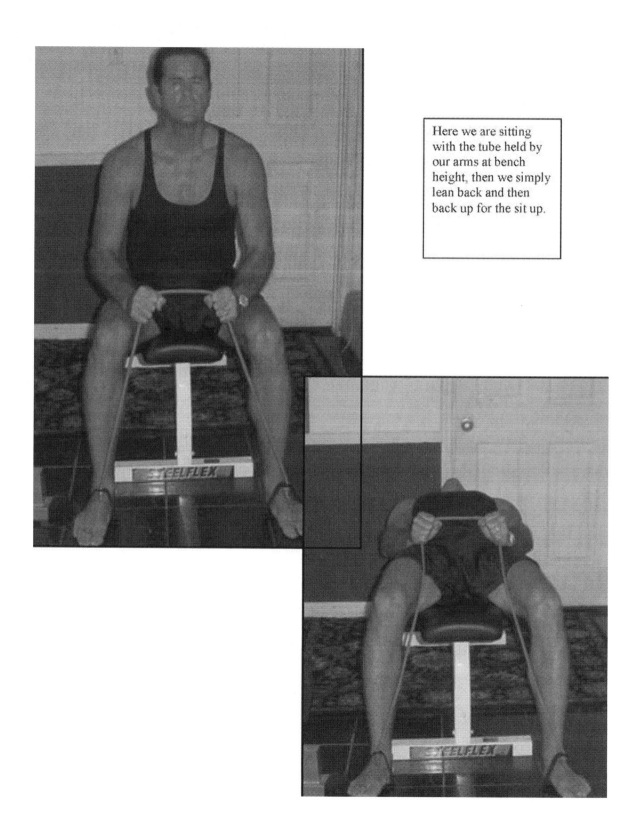

Here we are sitting with the tube held by our arms at bench height, then we simply lean back and then back up for the sit up.

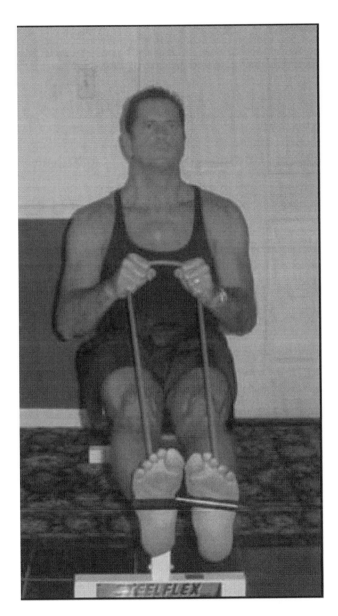

Here we are sitting with the tube held by our arms and around the feet, the feet are extended in front of the body, then we do our sit ups.

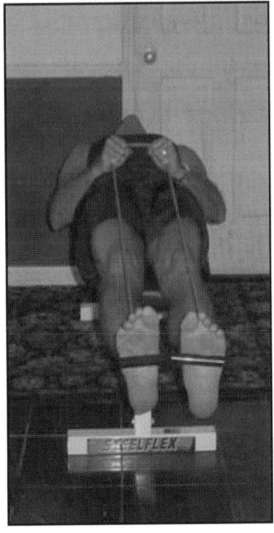

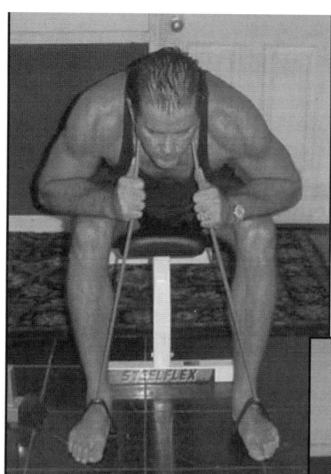

Here we are sitting with the tube held by our arms around the neck, while we are bent forward, then we sit up.

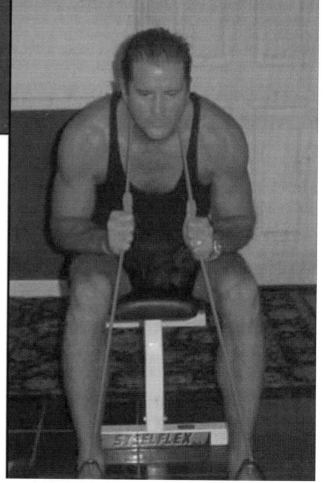

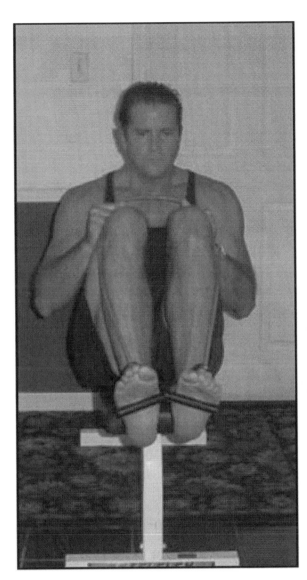

Here we work the lower abs by holding the tube with our feet, keeping or legs pulled in to the body, then extended out for the move. .

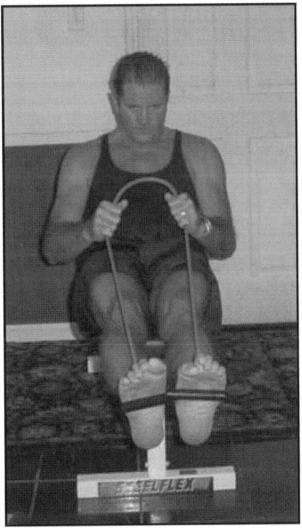

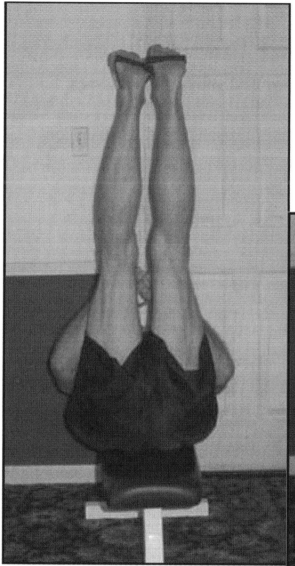

This a leg lift using the tube held by our feet. Simply lift the legs up and then down. .

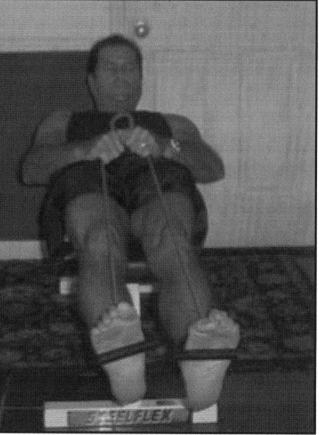

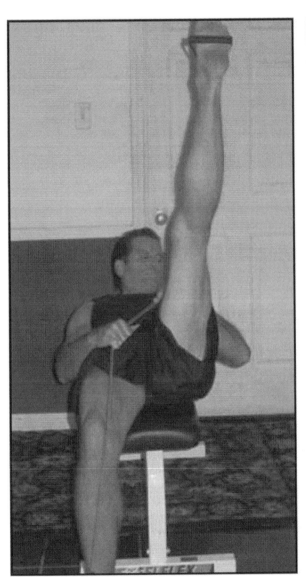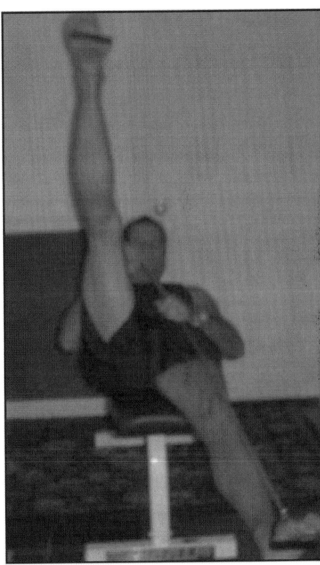

This is a variation of the leg lift were we alternate legs, first lifting one then the other. .

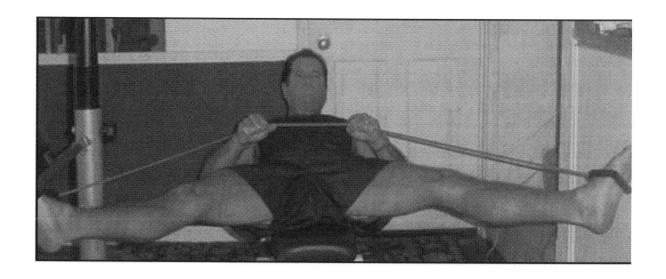

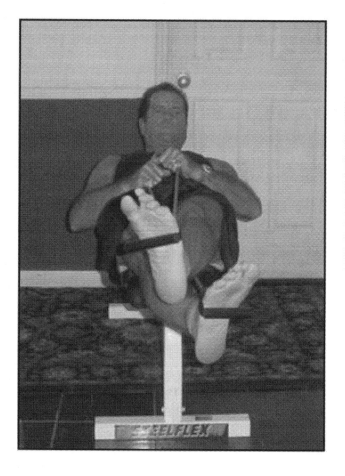

Here we start with the legs out fully extended to the side, then we being them together and over each other, alternating which leg goes on top with each movement. .

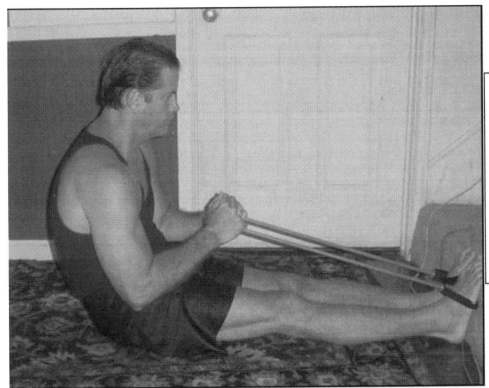

This is a sit up with the legs holding the tube and held against a wall for support, then we simply lean back and the up. .

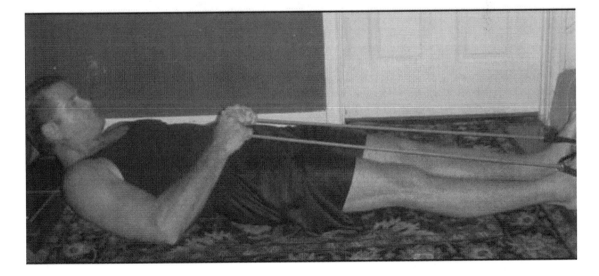

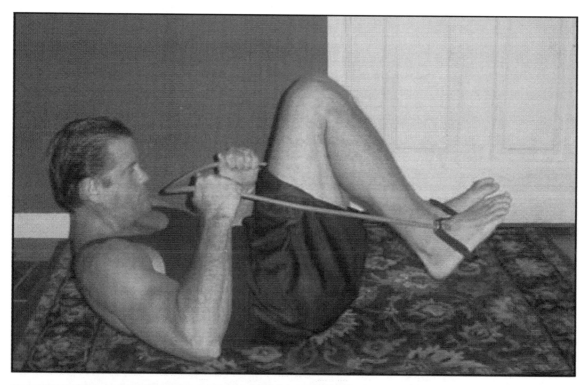

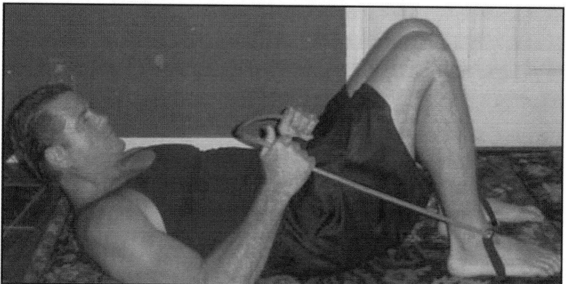

This is a modified crunch were we start with the legs bent holding the tube and then extend them down to the ground. .

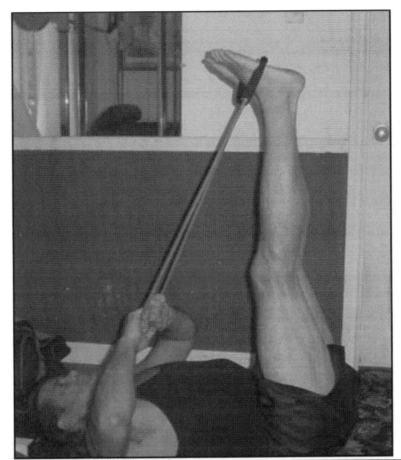

This is a leg lift starting with the legs directly up in front of the body then letting the fall down to the front, but not letting them touch the ground before coming back up. .

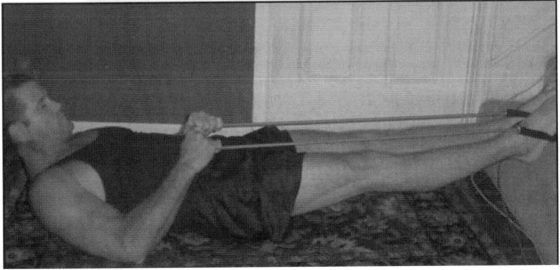

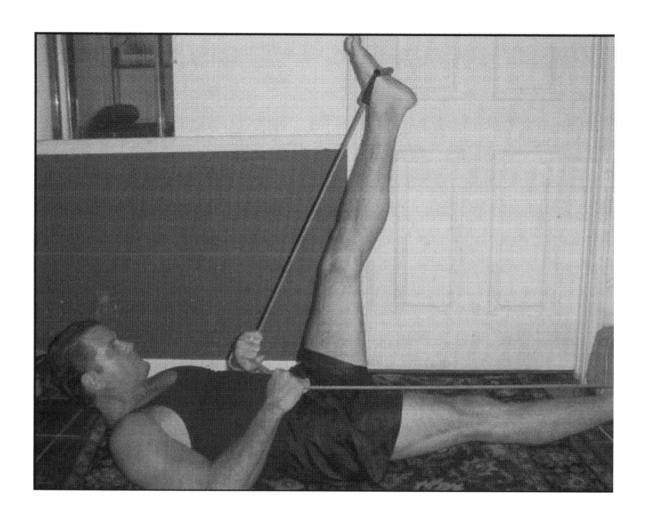

Here we are doing a leg scissor
with one leg up and then we bring it
down to the front.

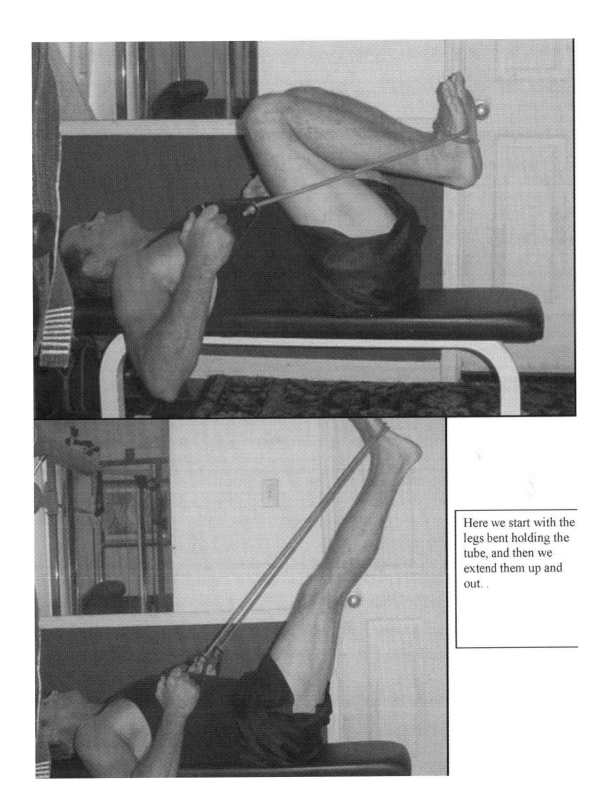

Here we start with the legs bent holding the tube, and then we extend them up and out. .

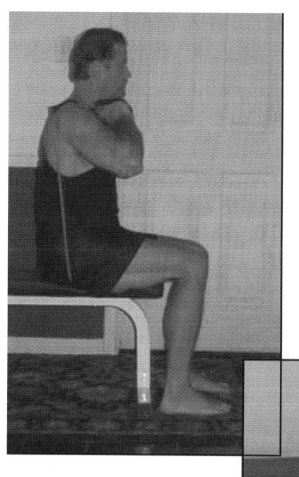

This is a sit down, we hold the tube up across our shoulders by sitting one it, then we simply lean down and forward to do the move.

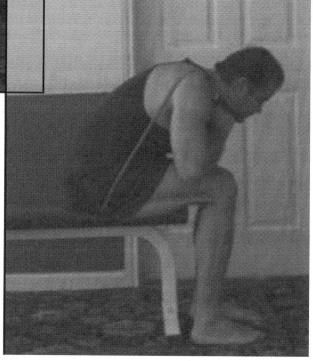

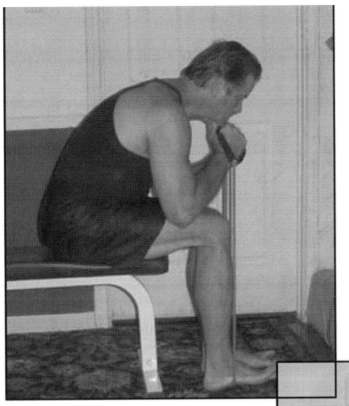

This is a sit back, we
hold the tube to our
chin, while leaning
down, then the we pull
our body up straight. .

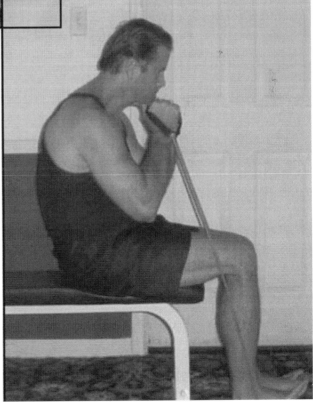

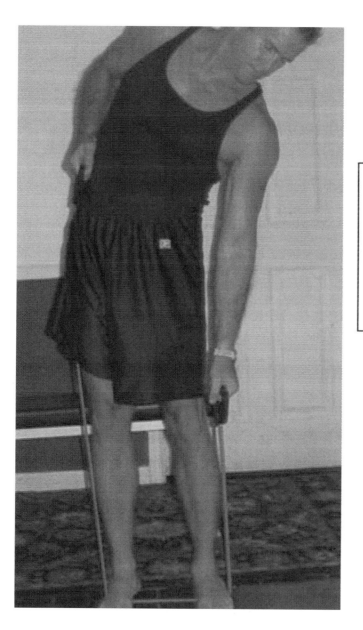

This moves work the love handles. We hold the tube with our feet and alternate leaning down and to the side. .

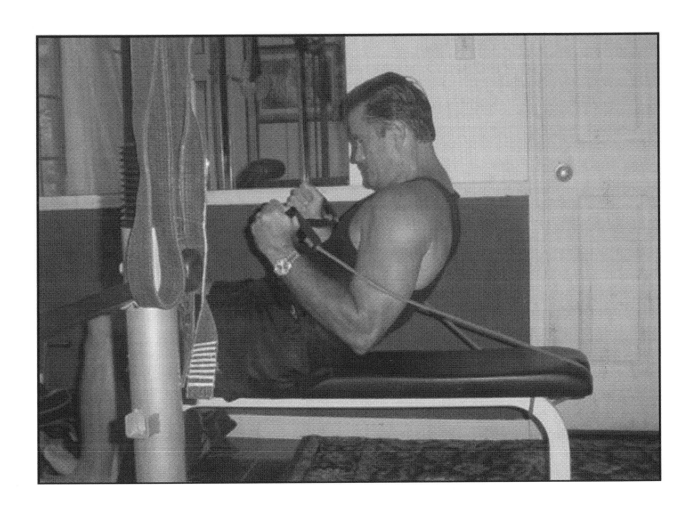

This is a sit up done
with the tube wrapped
around the back of the
bench.

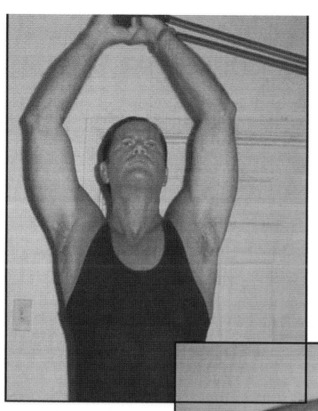

This move will work our love handles. Holding the tube high over head with both hand we lean to the sides, alternating sides. .

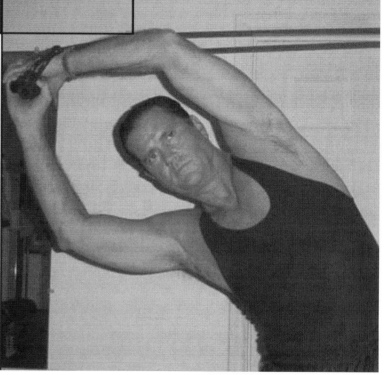

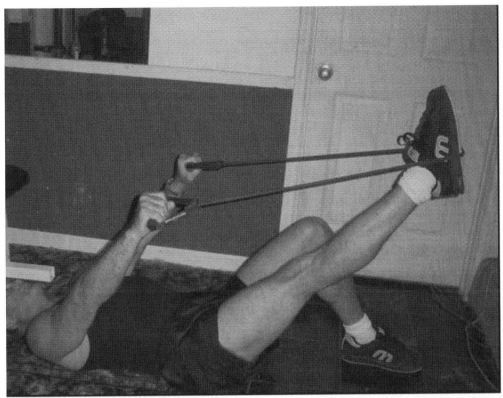

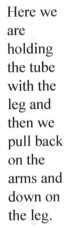

Here we are holding the tube with the leg and then we pull back on the arms and down on the leg.

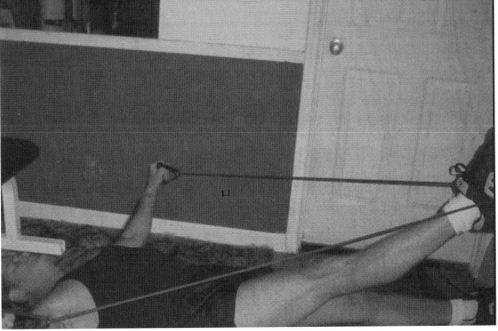

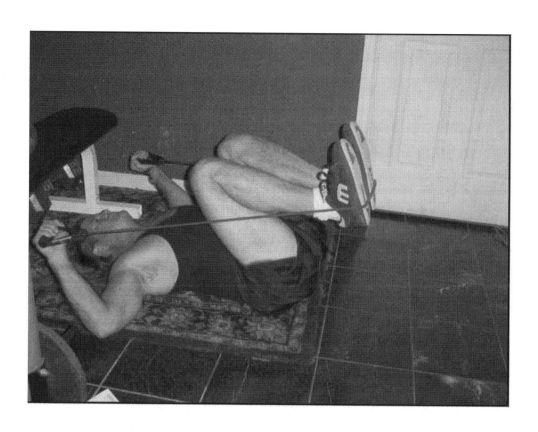

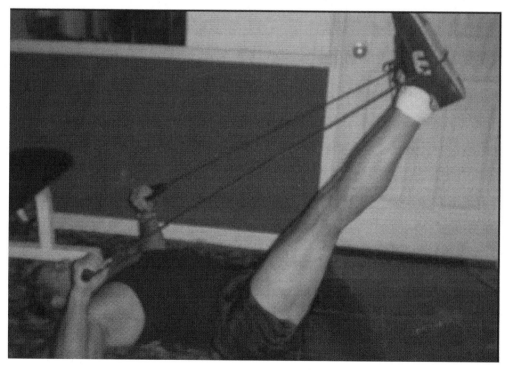

Arm Exercises

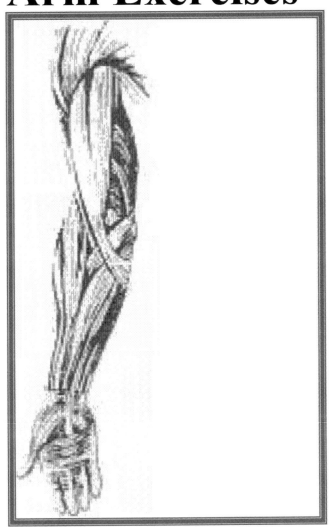

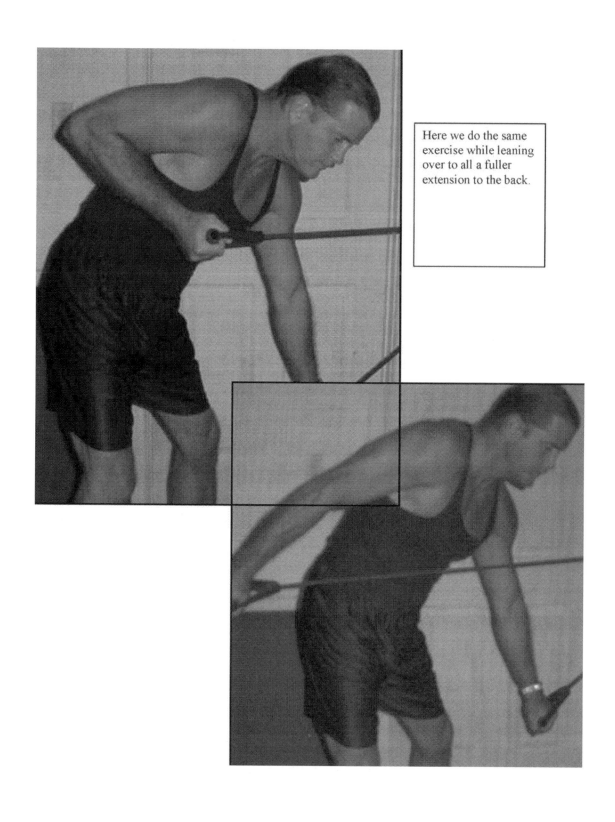

Here we do the same exercise while leaning over to all a fuller extension to the back.

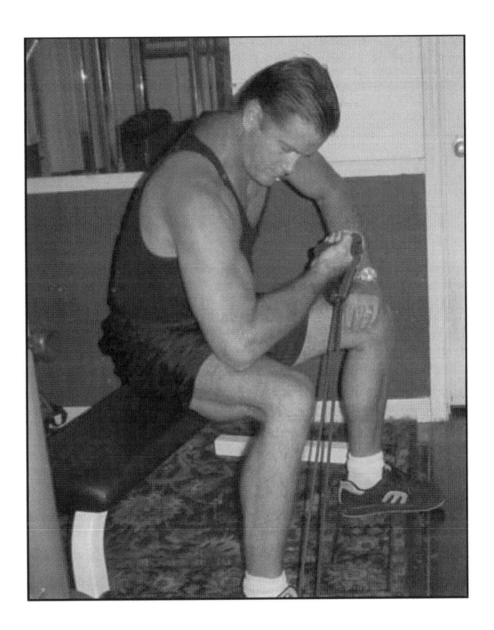

Here we work the
biceps by sitting down
and having the arm sit
on top of our knee then
pulling the arm up.

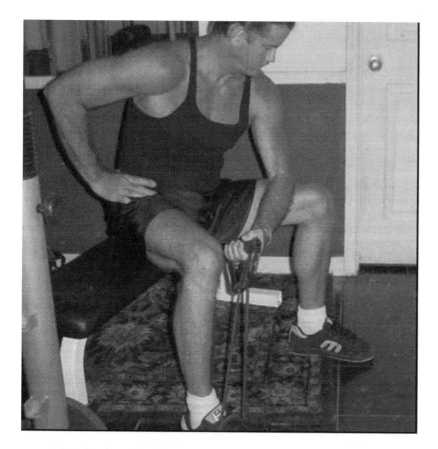

Here we work the biceps sitting down with the arm on top of our knee, then lifting up to the chest.

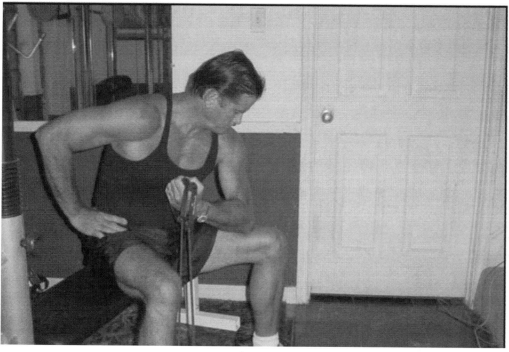

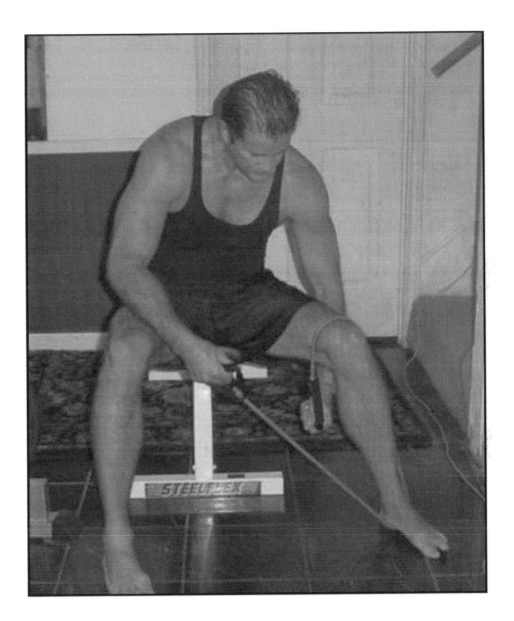

Here I show how to
wrap the tube around
my leg for exercising.

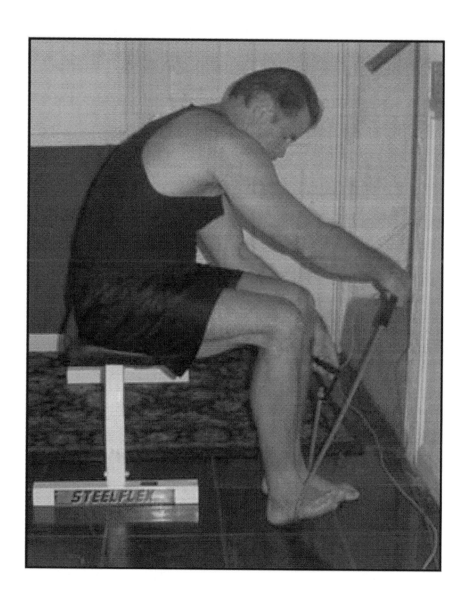

Here I show how to wrap the feet
around the tube for exercising.

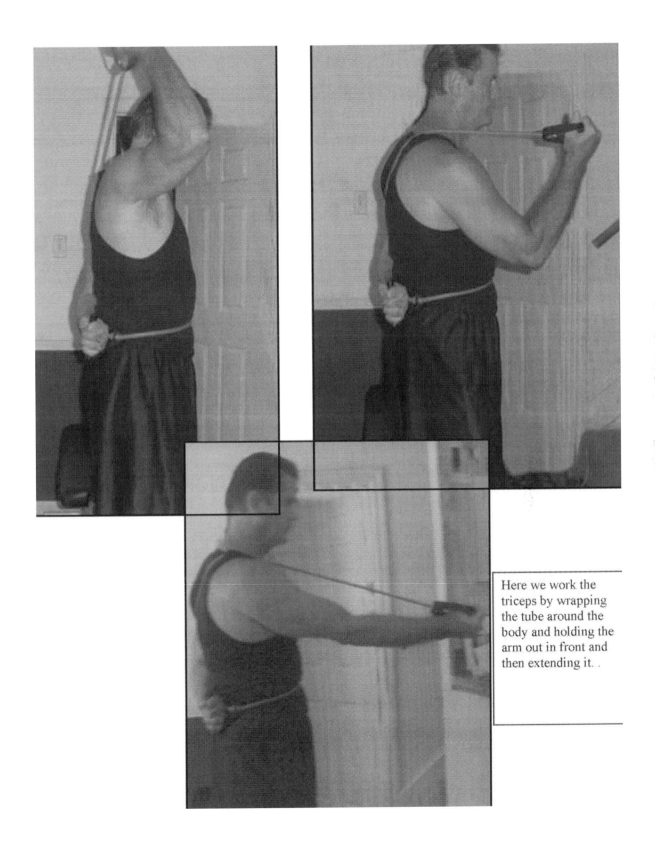

Here we work the triceps by wrapping the tube around the body and holding the arm out in front and then extending it. .

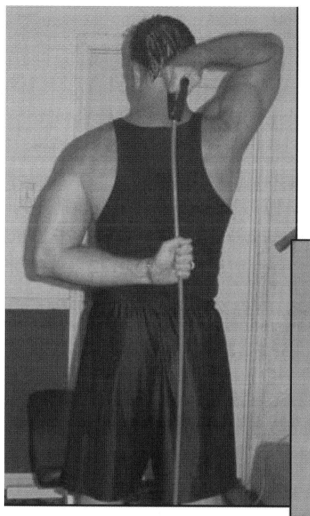

Here we work the tricep holding the tube behind our back and then extending the arm up. .

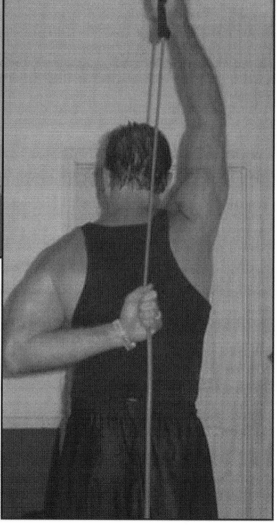

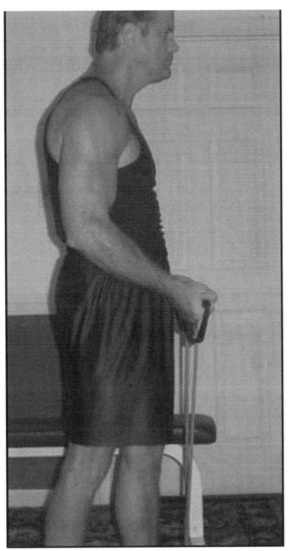

Here do a standing
double bicep curl.

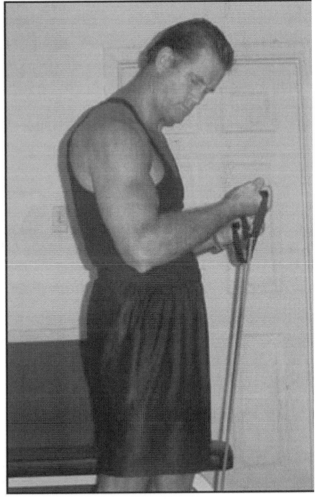

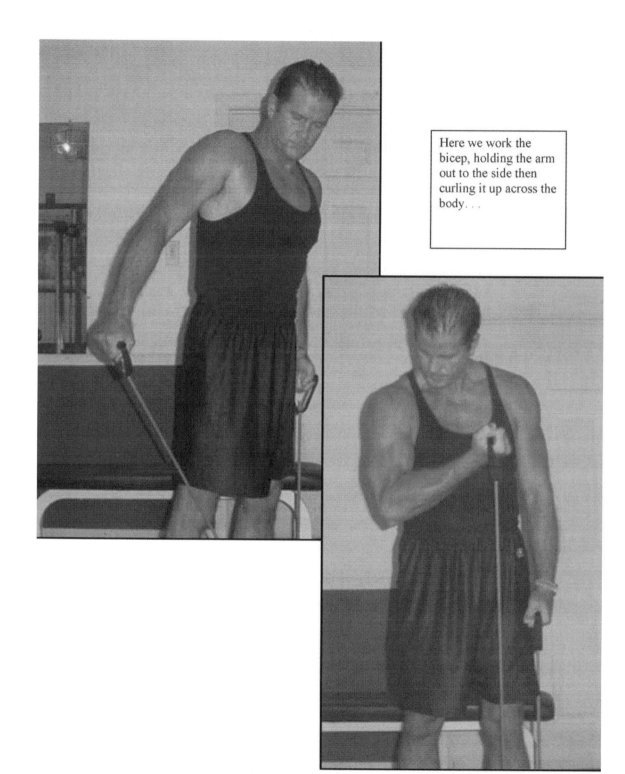

Here we work the bicep, holding the arm out to the side then curling it up across the body. . .

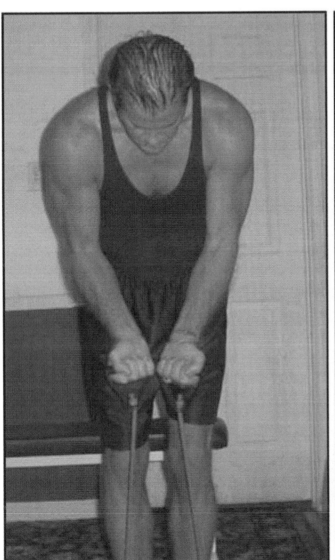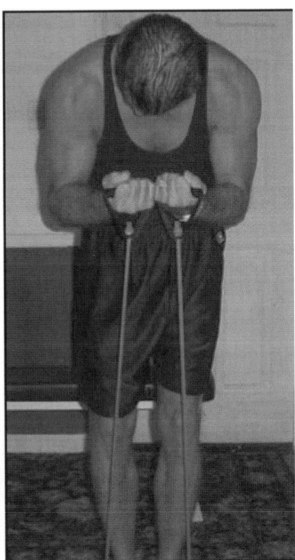

Here we work biceps bending over holding the tube with both hand and then curling up. .

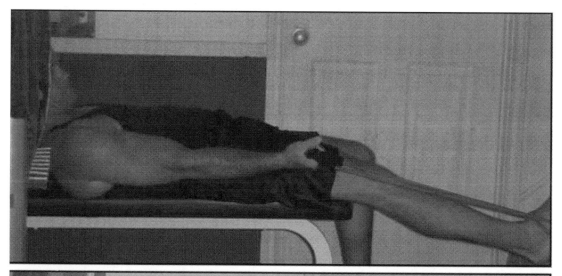

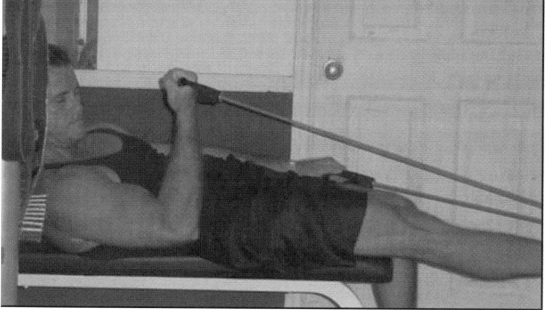

Here we work biceps lying
down on the bench and
extending the leg to hold the
tube and give more resistance
as we do the curl. .

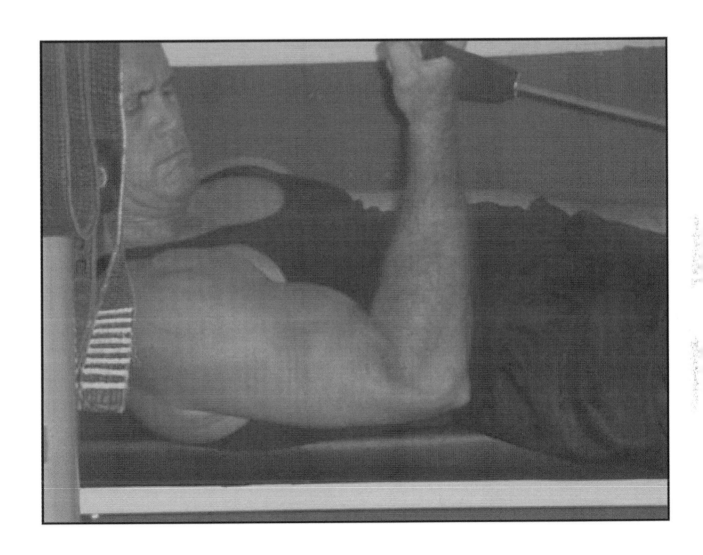

To get the most effect
from the exercise
really concentrate the
mind of the muscle
you are working. .

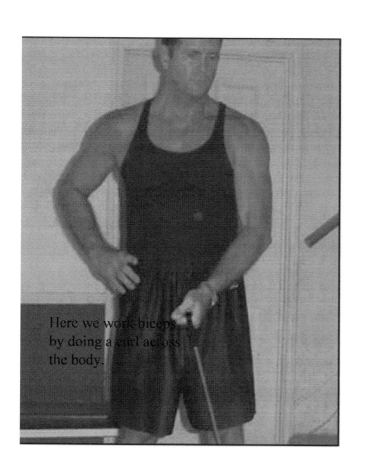

Here we work biceps by doing a curl across the body.

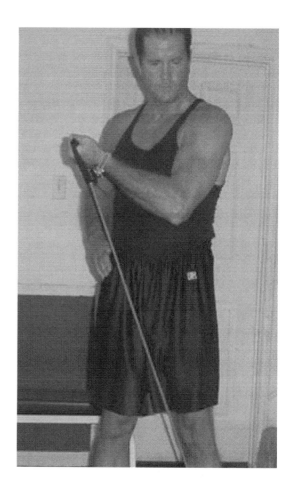

Chest Exercises

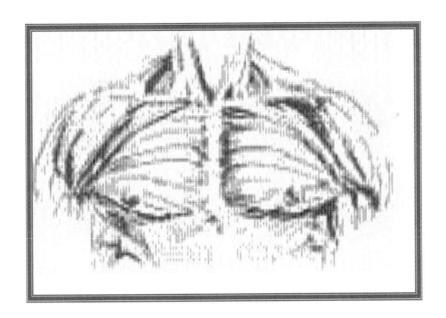

One Arm Chest

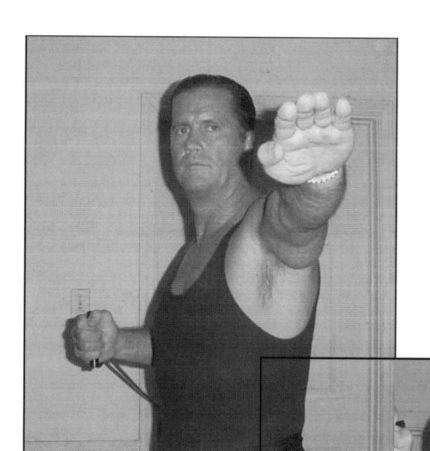

This is a easy exercise to work the Chest. Simply twist the body forward while extending the arm directly at chest height.

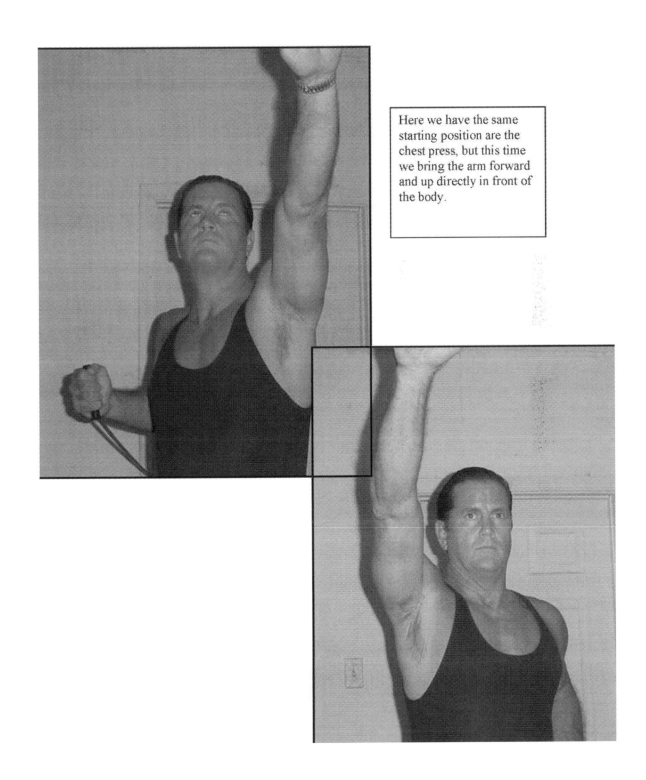

Here we have the same starting position are the chest press, but this time we bring the arm forward and up directly in front of the body.

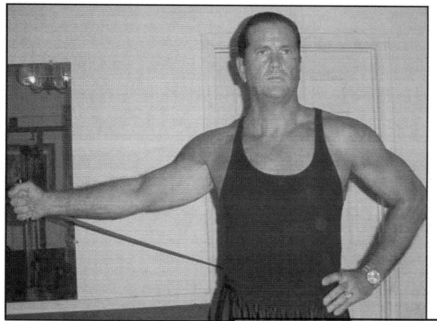

Here we start with the arm directly out to the side of the chest and bring the arm across the body and in front to work the lower chest.

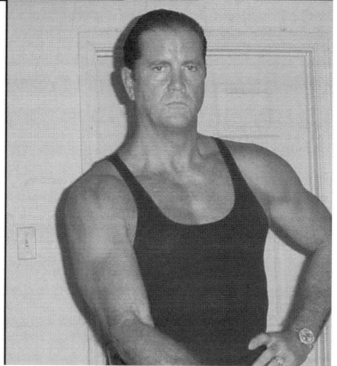

Here we start with the arm directly out to the side of the chest and bring the arm across the body and in front to work the lower chest.

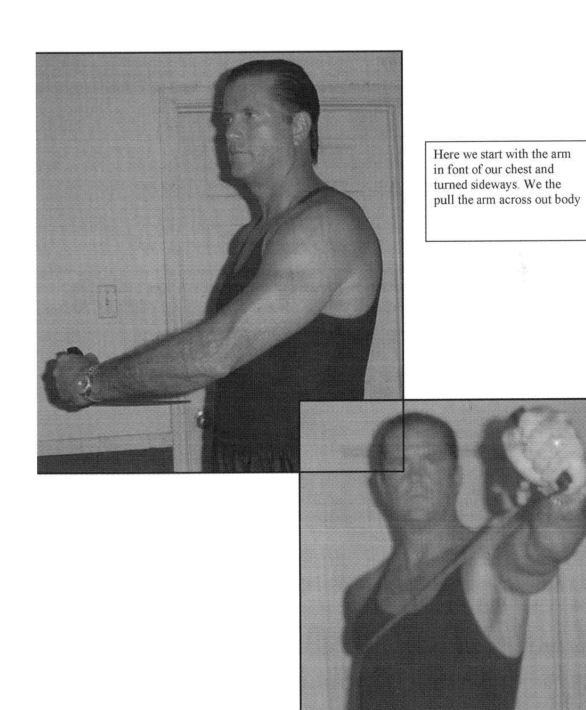

Here we start with the arm in font of our chest and turned sideways. We the pull the arm across out body

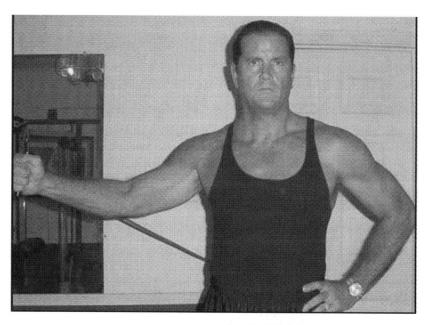

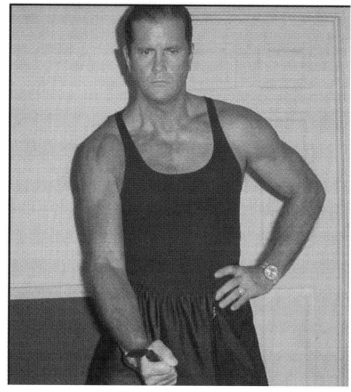

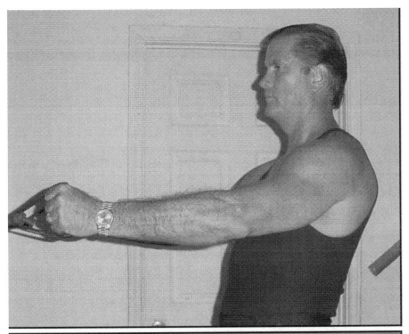

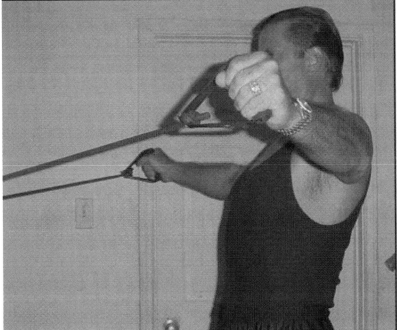

Here we hold the tube directly in front of the body with the palms facing up, then we pull the arms back and to the sides.

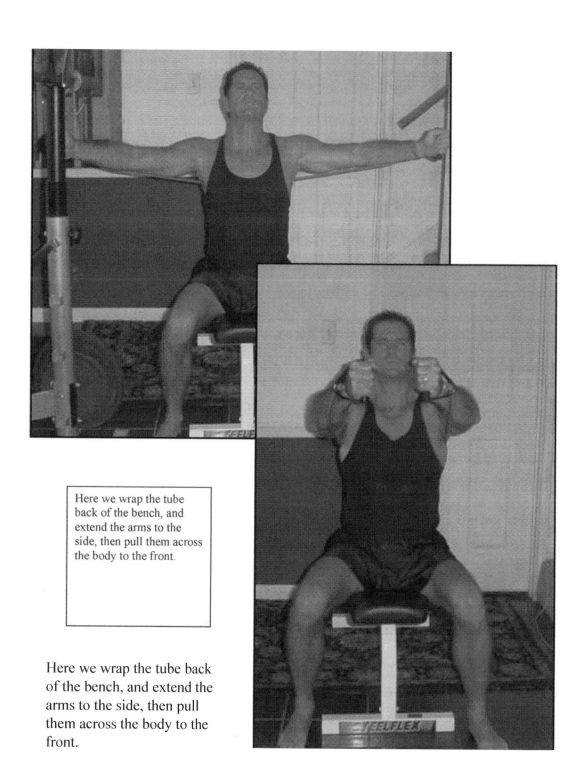

Here we wrap the tube
back of the bench, and
extend the arms to the
side, then pull them across
the body to the front.

Here we wrap the tube back
of the bench, and extend the
arms to the side, then pull
them across the body to the
front.

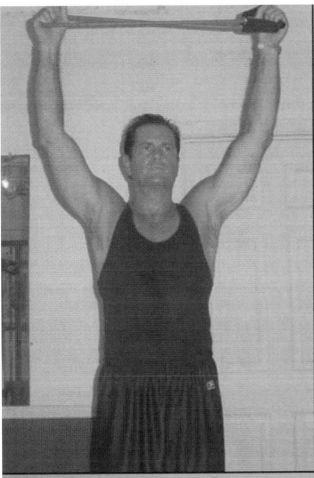

Here we hold the tube up over the head with the arms extended and then pull the arms down until they are at shoulder height.

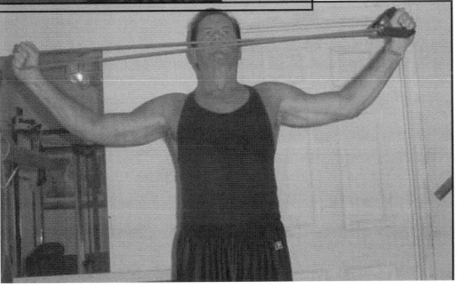

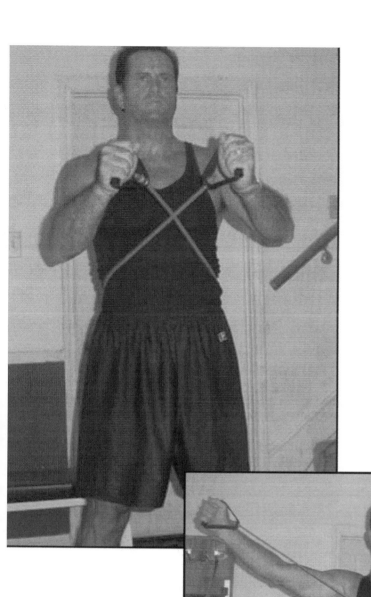

Here we wrap the tube around the body, crossing it in front, then pull the arms directly apart.

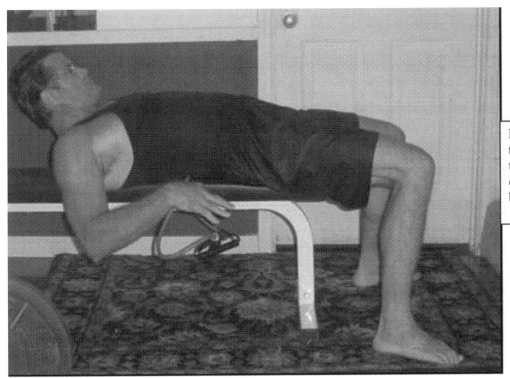

Here we wrap the tube under the bench and do a regular bench press.

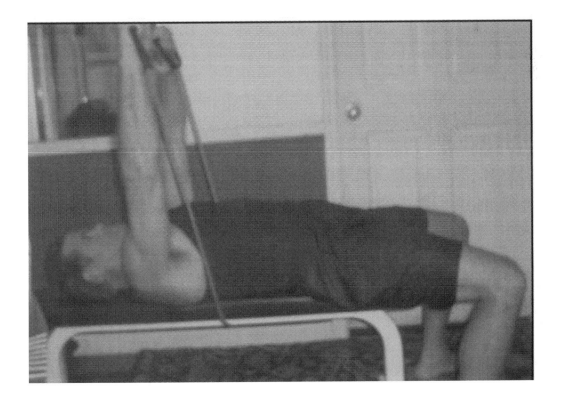

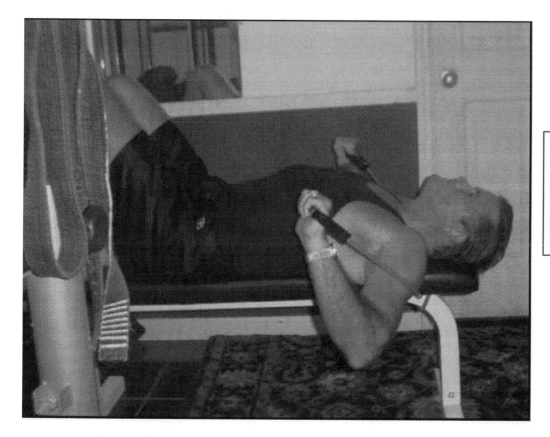

Here we wrap the tube under the do a bench press forward and out to work the lower chest. .

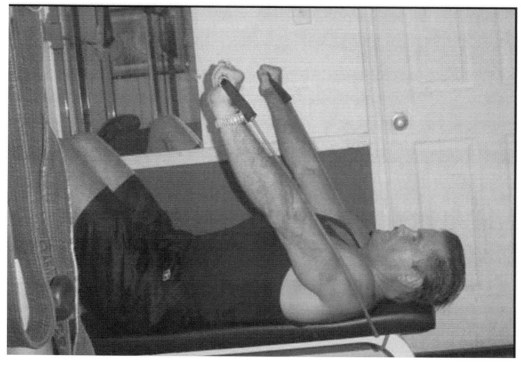

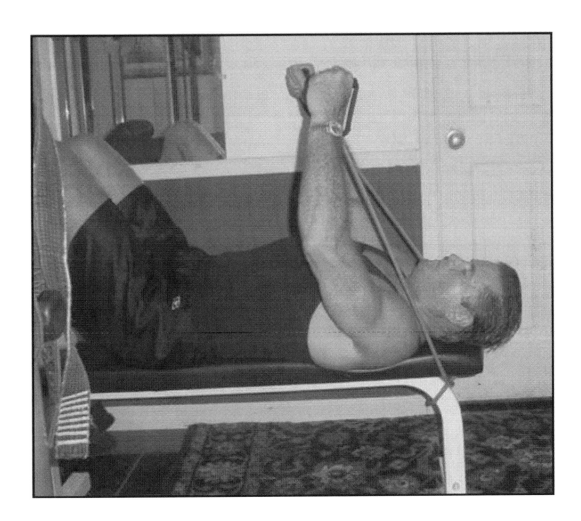

Here we wrap the tube
under the bench and do
a regular bench press.,
but this time we cross
the tube in front of our
body.

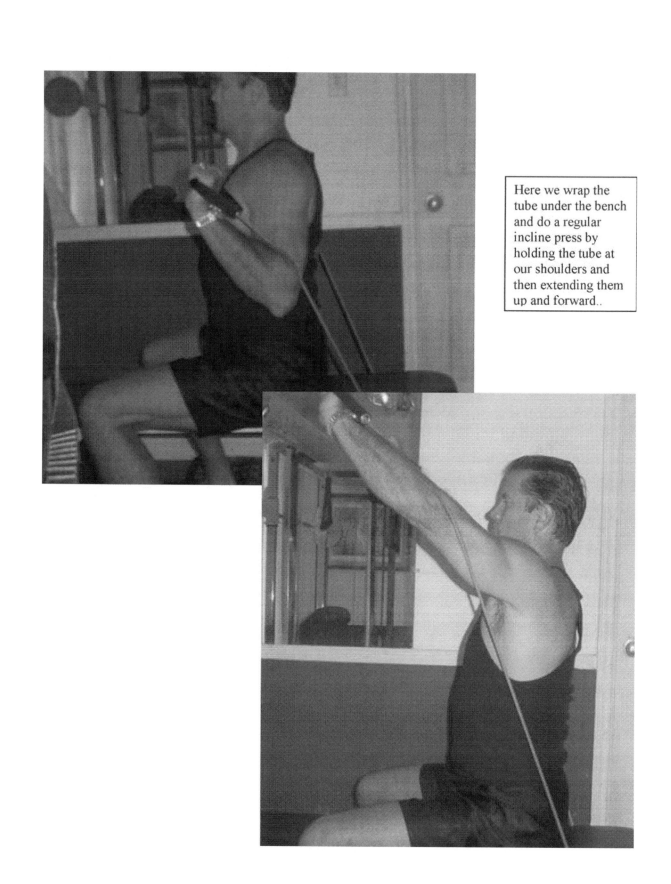

Here we wrap the tube under the bench and do a regular incline press by holding the tube at our shoulders and then extending them up and forward..

Leg Exercises

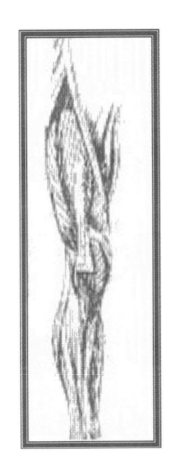

Here we do a basic
squat by holding the
tube at shoulder height,
locked under our feet,
then we sit down and
back up. Be sure to
keep the back straight
and the head up.

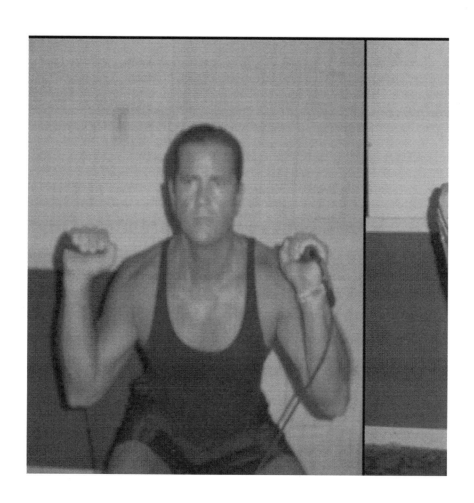

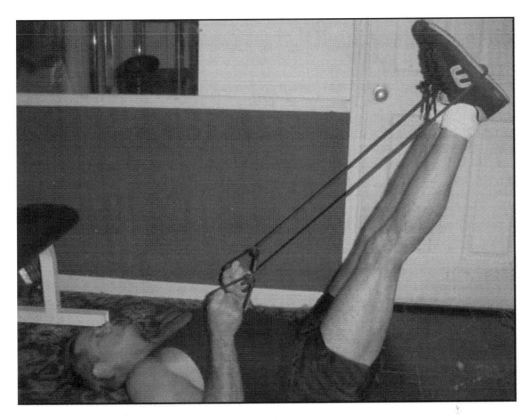

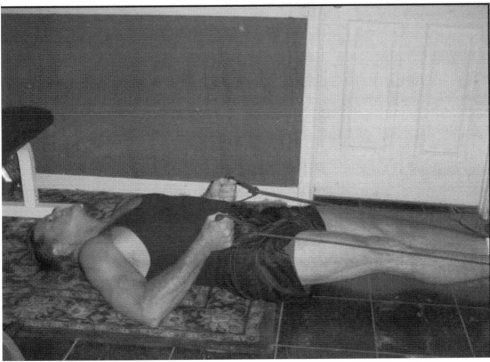

Here we work the legs by holding the tube up with the feet and then bring it down to the ground.

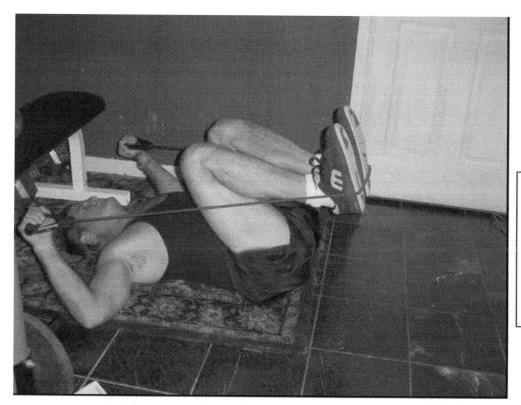

Here we work the legs by holding the tube with the feet and the legs bent, then extending the legs up and out.

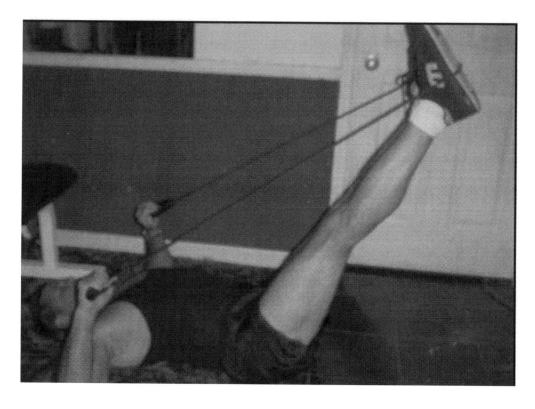

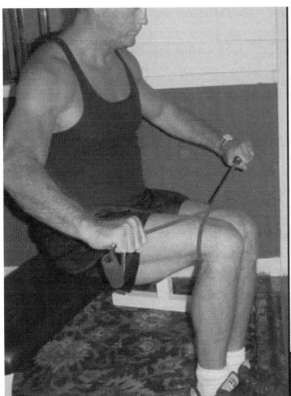

Here we work the inner thigh by wrapping the tube around knees the pulling the legs apart at the knees.

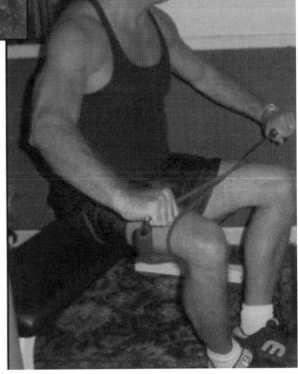

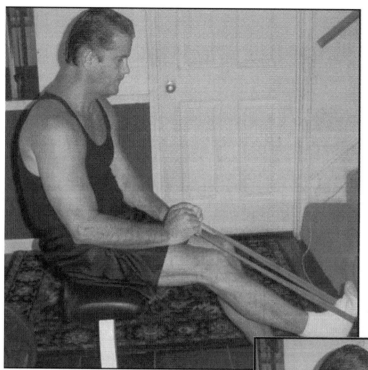

Here we hold
the tube on
our foot work
the ankle and
calf, by
extending the
ankle.

This is the same
exercise done
without a sock for
a more secure
hold.

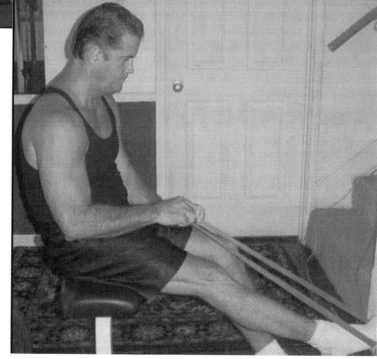

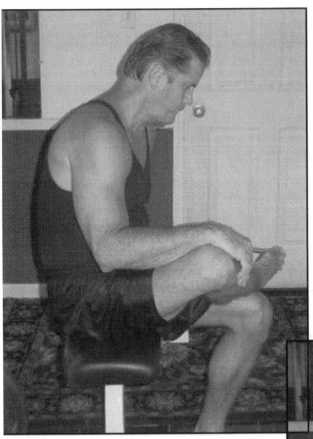

Here we work
the ankle by
wrapping the
tube around
the foot and
then flexing it.

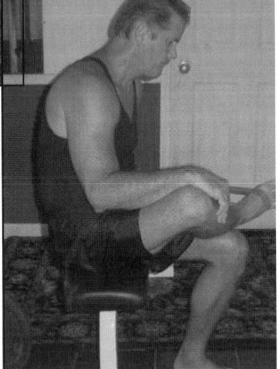

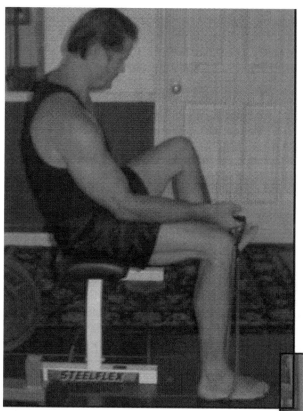

Here we hold the tube wrapped around out foot and held by the other foot with the leg bent, then we extend the foot forward.

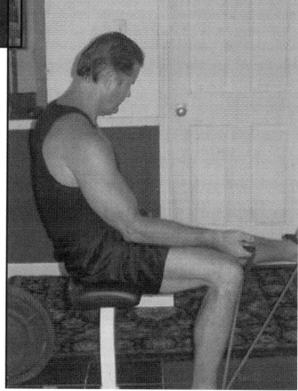

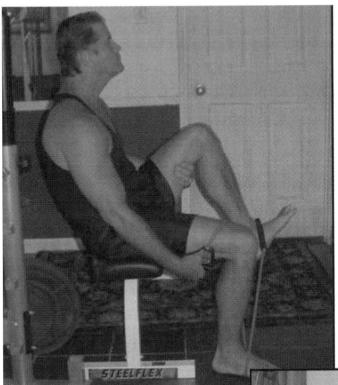

Here we hold the tube wrapped around out foot and held by the other foot with the leg bent, then we extend the foot forward. We hold the extending leg for support.

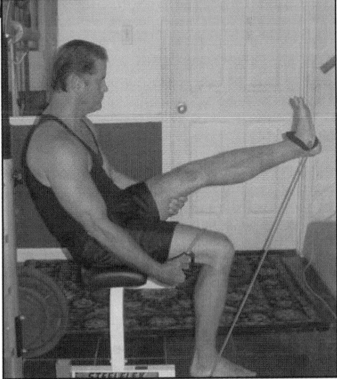

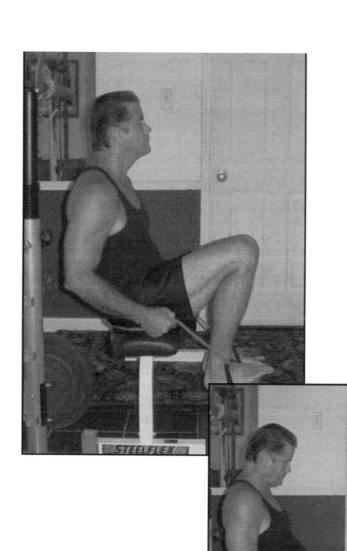

Here we hold the ends of the tube with both feet and then extend the legs forward.

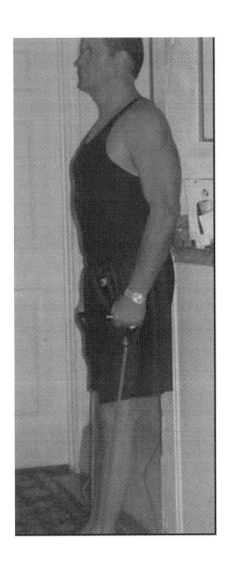

Here we do a squat with our back to the wall for support, while standing on the tube.

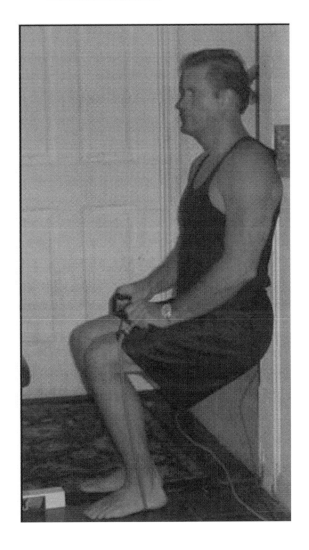

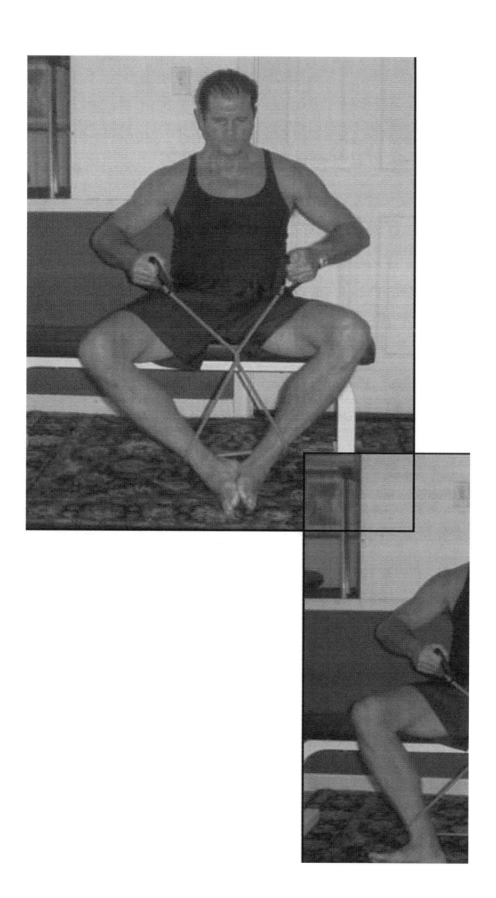

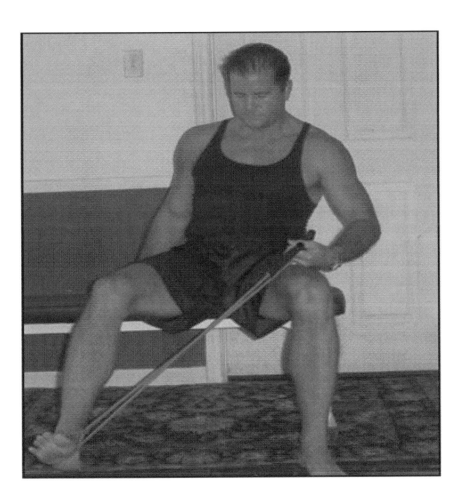

Here wrap the tube over the foot and pull the leg away from the bench.

Here we wrap the
tube around the
foot and pull the
leg up and then
straight and then
out.

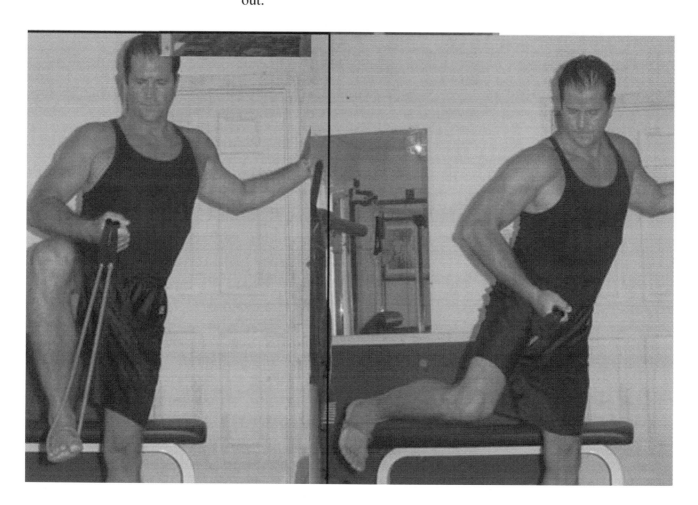

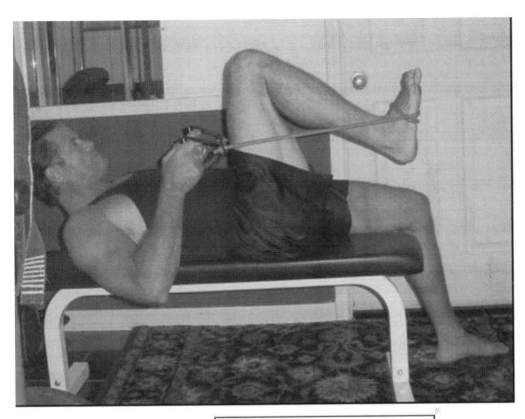

Here wrap the tube around the foot, bending the leg and then extending it directly out.

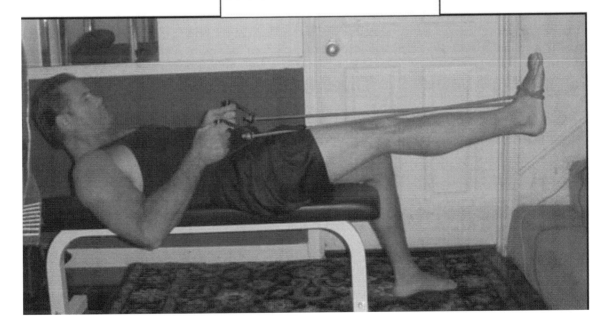

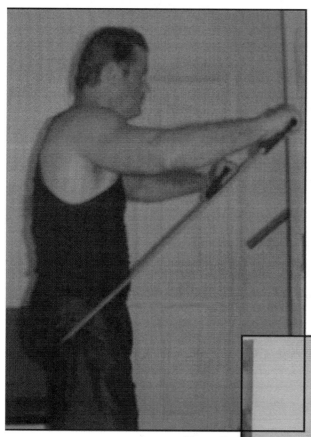

Here we do a modified squat by wrapping the tube around our hips and then sitting up and down. Keep the elbows wide and out.

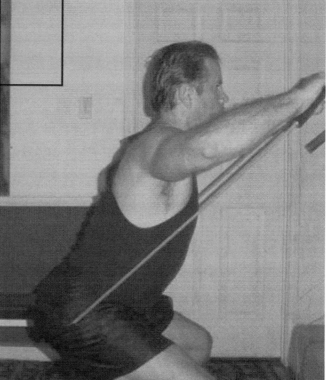

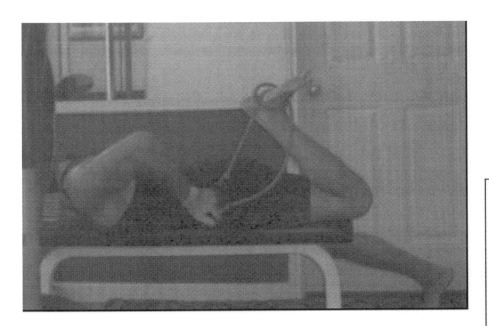

Here we wrap the tube around our foot, while lying face down on the bench, then extend the leg out and back.

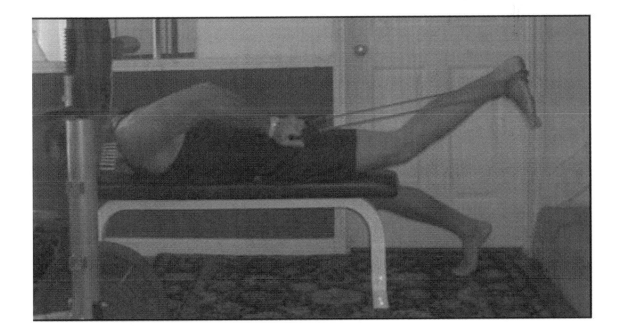

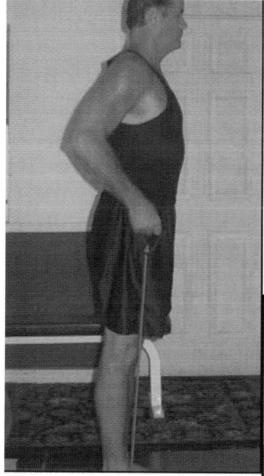

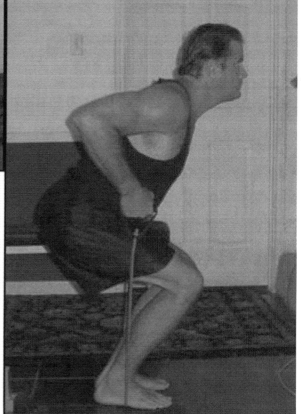

Here we do a squat by standing on the tube and bending down and then back up.

Here we hold the tube with our feet and while having the legs bent, then we extend them up and out.

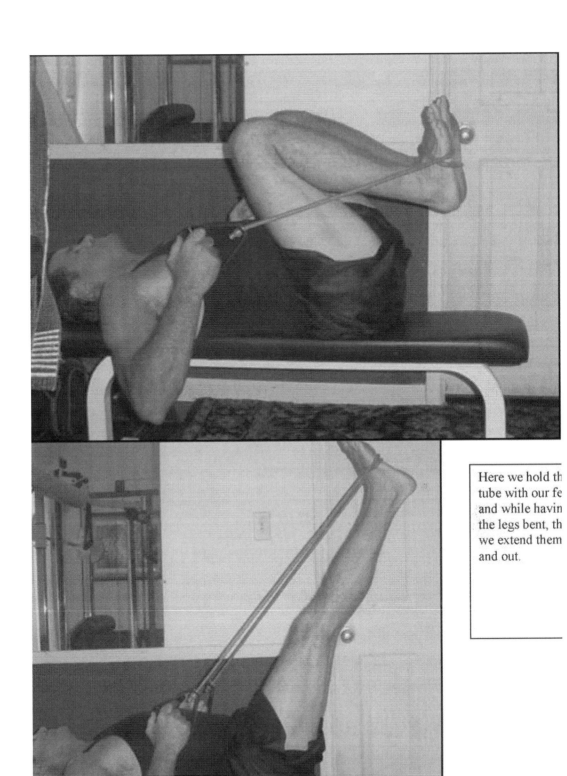

Here we hold th
tube with our fe
and while havin
the legs bent, th
we extend them
and out.

Lat Exercises

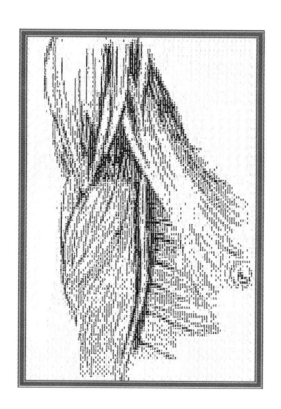

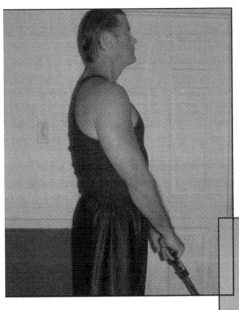

Here we work the lats by holding the tube out in front of the body then pulling it up and towards the back.

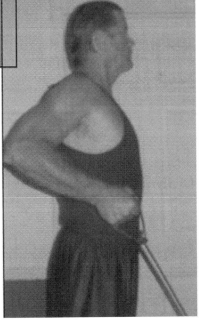

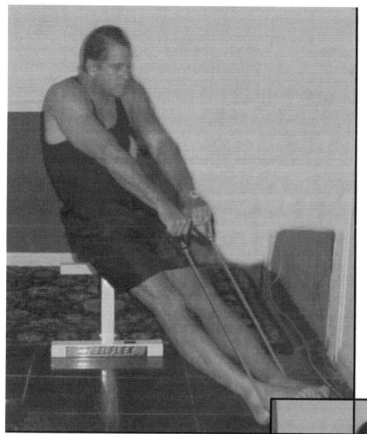

Here we work the lats holding the tube with the feet and the legs locked out in front of the body, lean slightly forward, and then we pull back with the arms

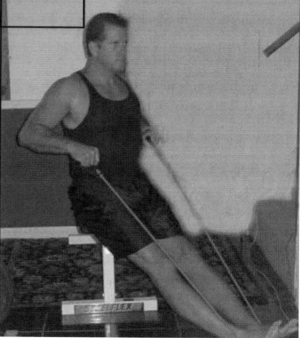

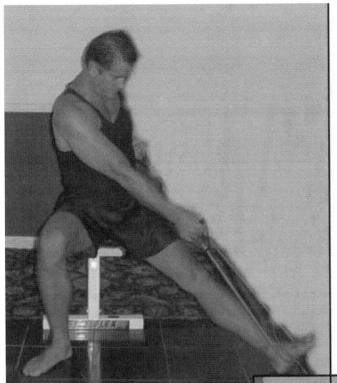

Here we work the lats extending the leg forward and holding the tube with the foot, then pulling back with one arm.

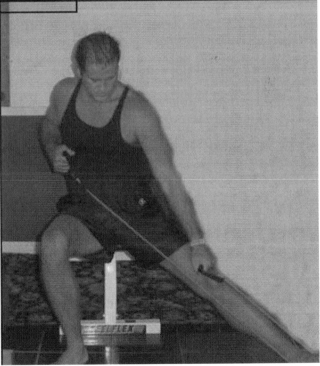

Here we work the
lats leaning forward
holding the tube
with both feet,

Here we work the
lats leaning
forward holding
the tube with both
feet, leaning
backwards and
pulling the arms to
the side.

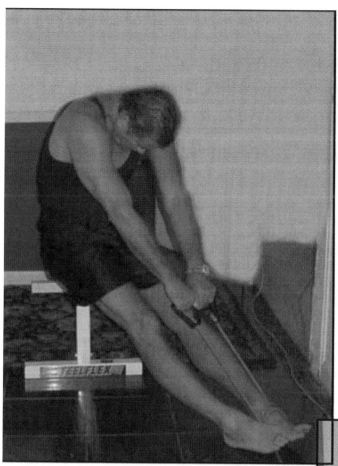

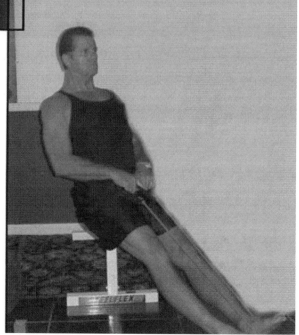

Martial Arts Exercises

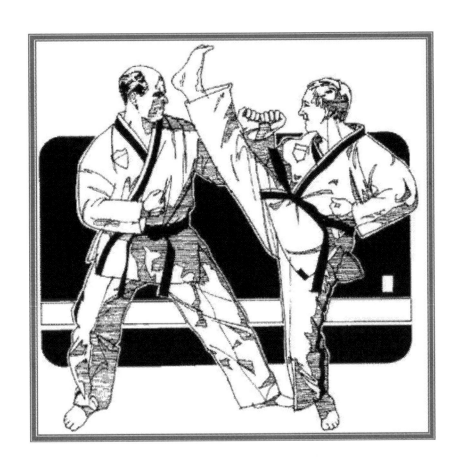

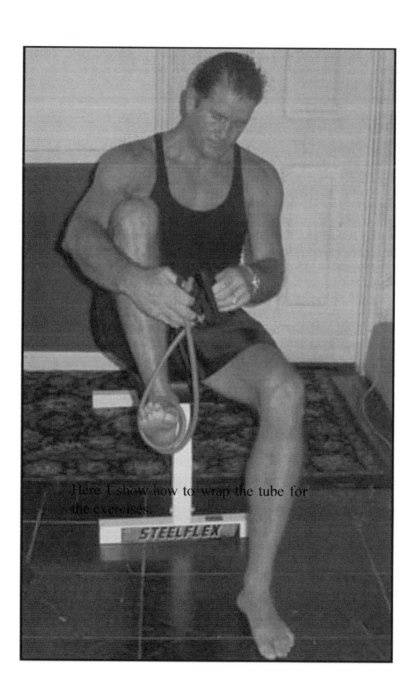

Here I show how to wrap the tube for the exercises.

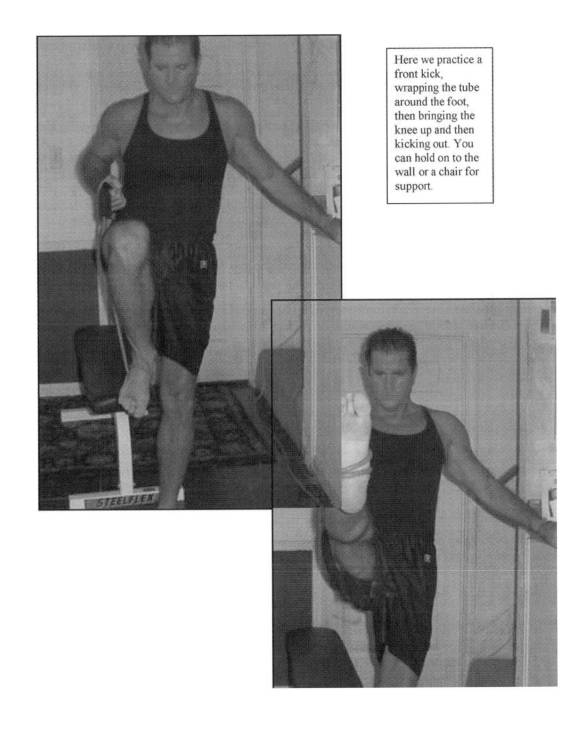

Here we practice a front kick, wrapping the tube around the foot, then bringing the knee up and then kicking out. You can hold on to the wall or a chair for support.

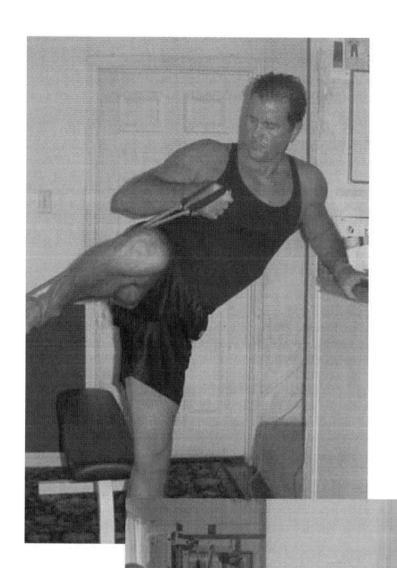

Here we practice a side kick, wrapping the tube around the foot, then bringing the knee up and then kicking out. You can hold on to the wall or a chair for support.

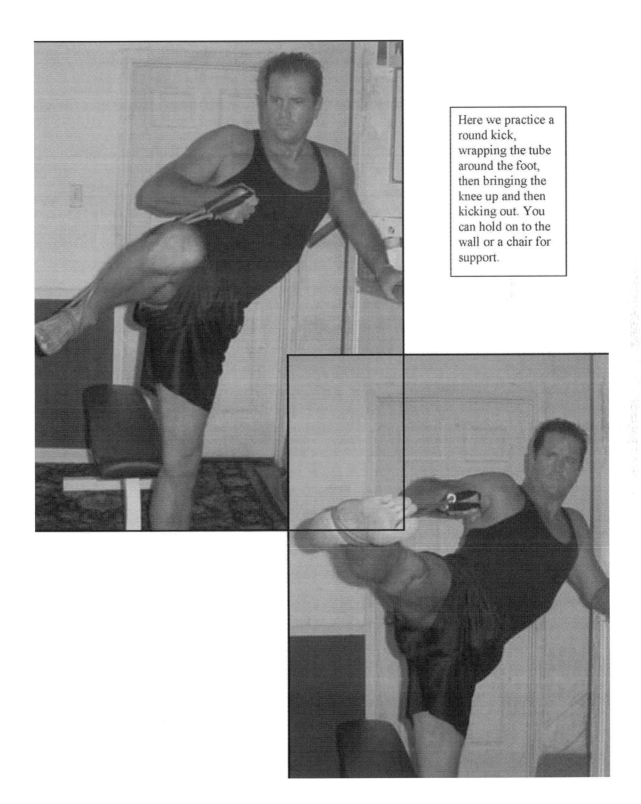

Here we practice a round kick, wrapping the tube around the foot, then bringing the knee up and then kicking out. You can hold on to the wall or a chair for support.

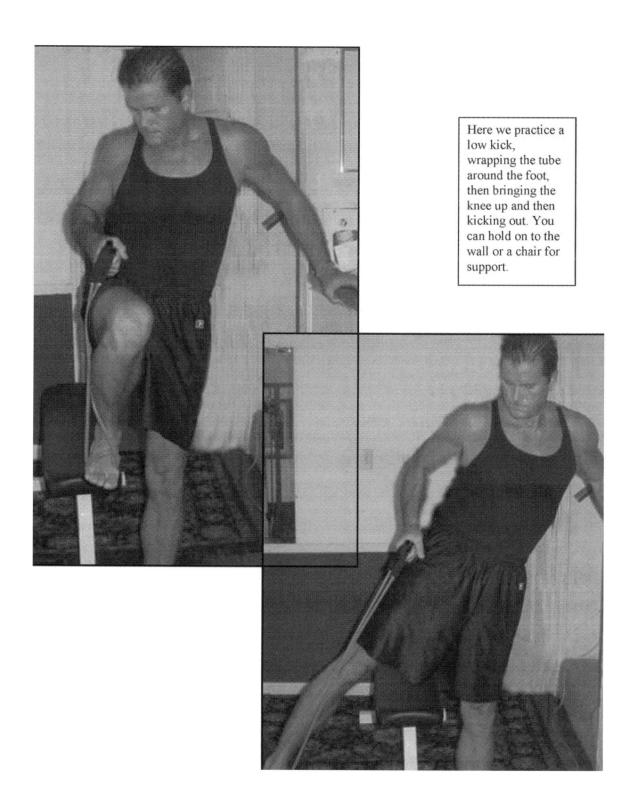

Here we practice a low kick, wrapping the tube around the foot, then bringing the knee up and then kicking out. You can hold on to the wall or a chair for support.

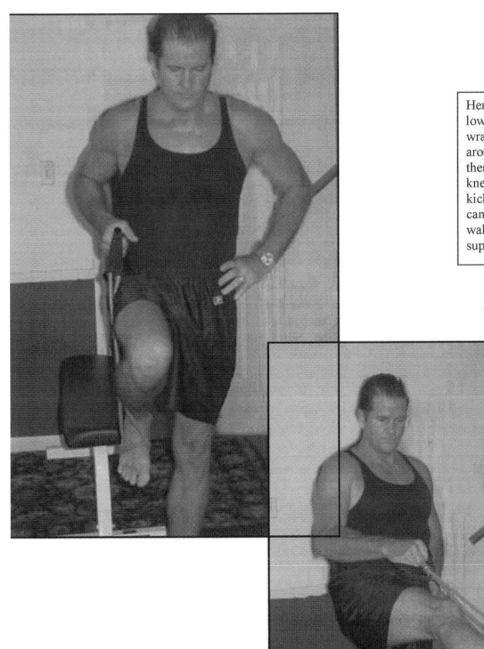

Here we practice a low front kick, wrapping the tube around the foot, then bringing the knee up and then kicking out. You can hold on to the wall or a chair for support.

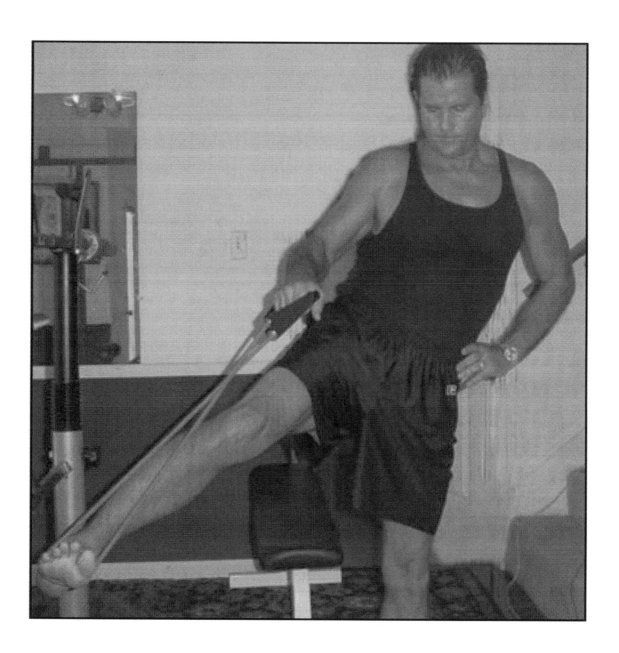

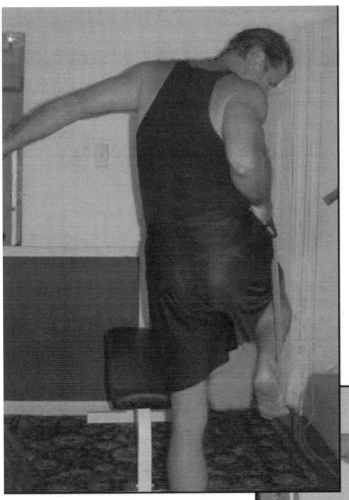

Here we practice a back kick, wrapping the tube around the foot, then bringing the knee up and then kicking out. You can hold on to the wall or a chair for support.

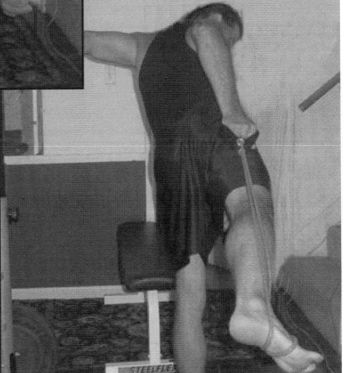

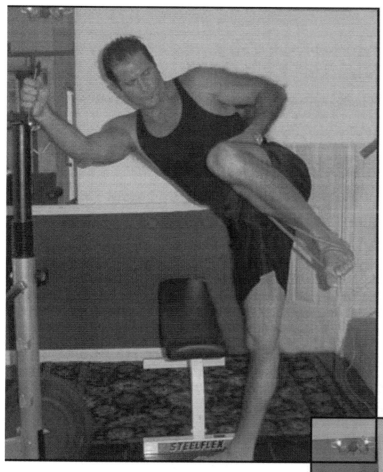

Here we practice a high round kick, wrapping the tube around the foot, then bringing the knee up and then kicking out. You can hold on to the wall or a chair for support.

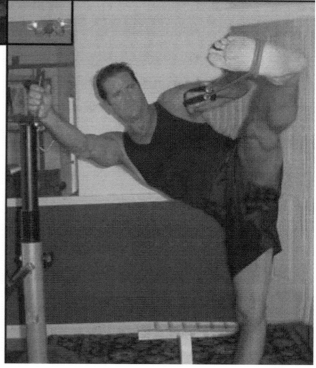

Here we practice a highest front kick, wrapping the tube around the foot, then bringing the knee up and then kicking out. You can hold on to the wall or a chair for support.

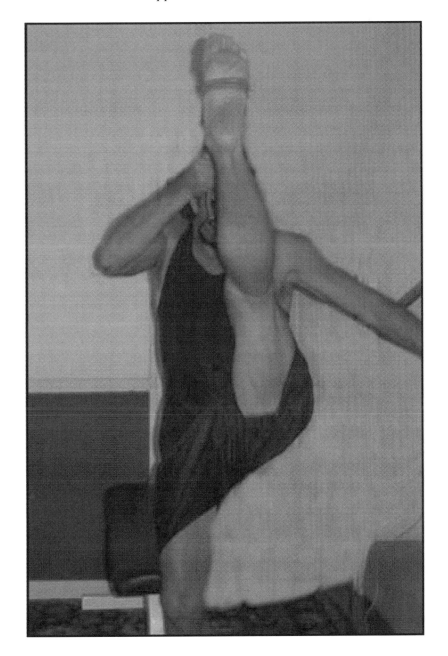

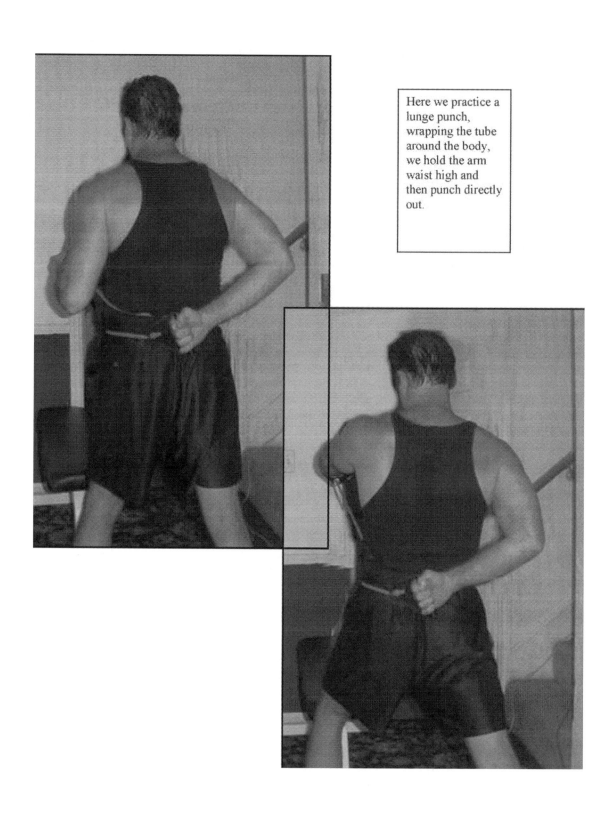

Here we practice a lunge punch, wrapping the tube around the body, we hold the arm waist high and then punch directly out.

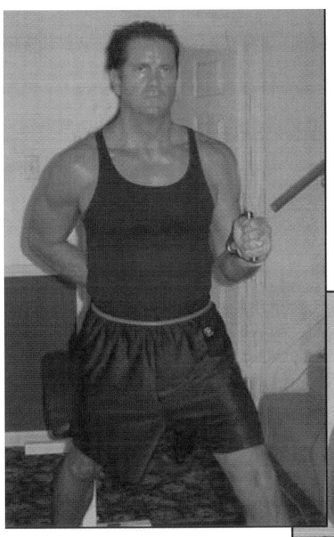

Here we practice a lunge punch, wrapping the tube around the body, we hold the arm waist high and then punch directly out.

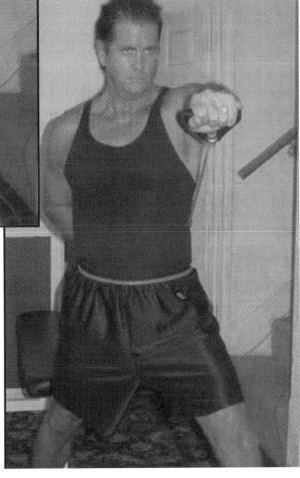

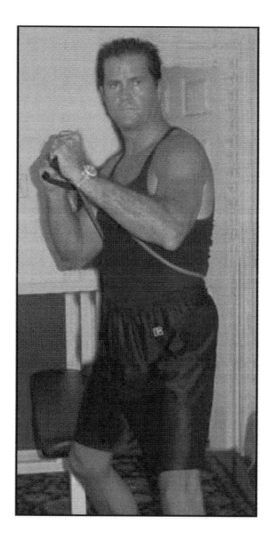

Here we practice a down block , wrapping the tube around the body, we hold arm up and in front, then snapping them down and back.

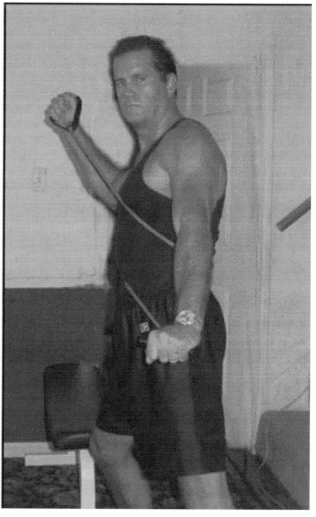

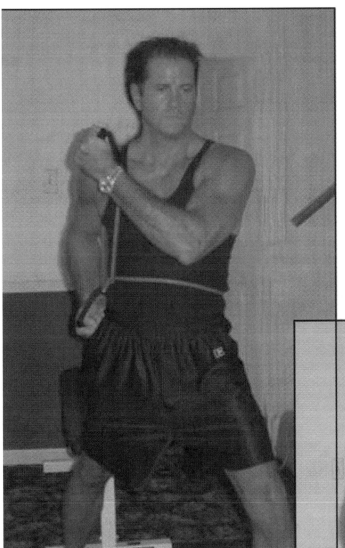

Here we practice a down block, holding one arm up in front of the body then twisting the body as we block down over the knee.

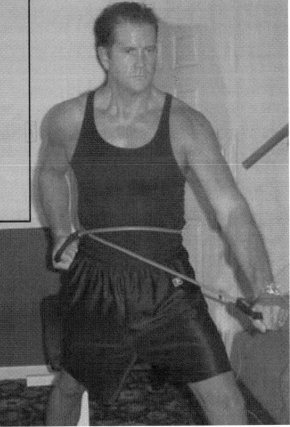

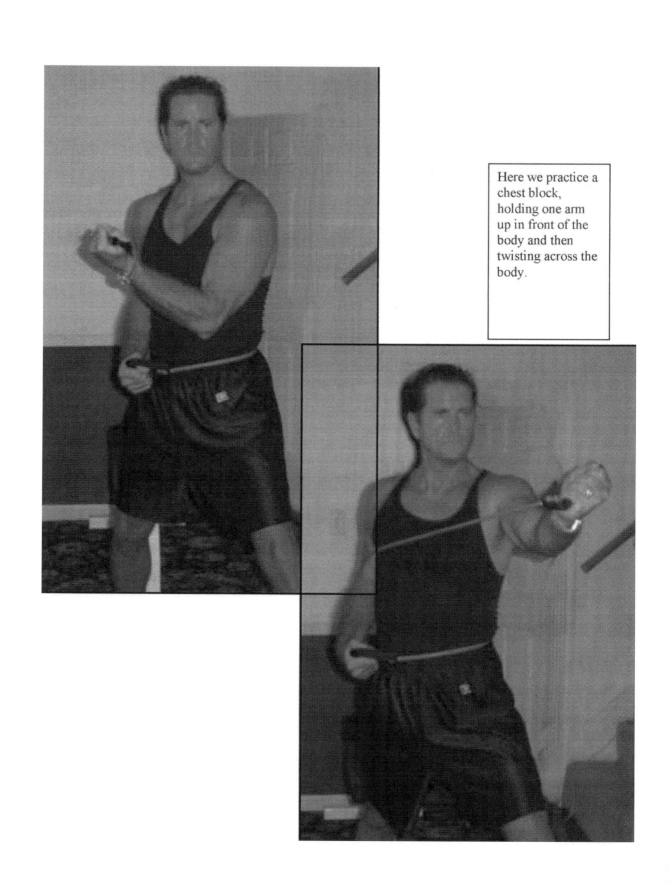

Here we practice a chest block, holding one arm up in front of the body and then twisting across the body.

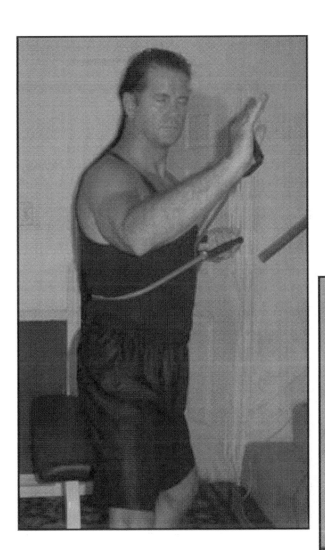

Here we practice a Knife hand block, holding one arm up in front of the body then snapping the arms across the body with the blade of the hand out.

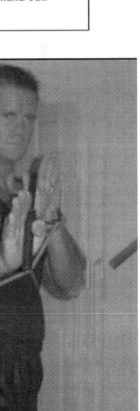

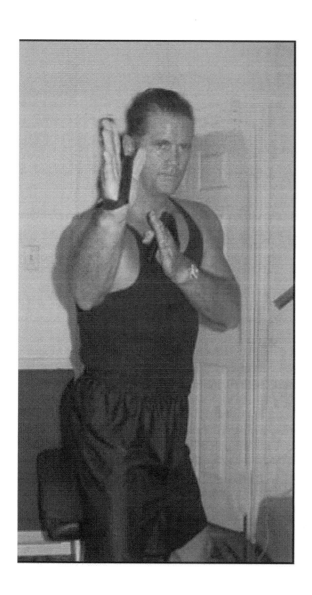

Here we practice a Knife hand block, holding one arm up in front of the body then snapping the arms across the body with the blade of the hand out and facing down.

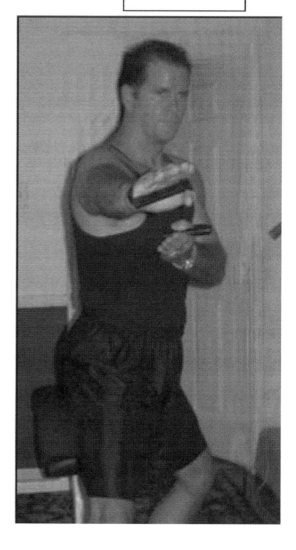

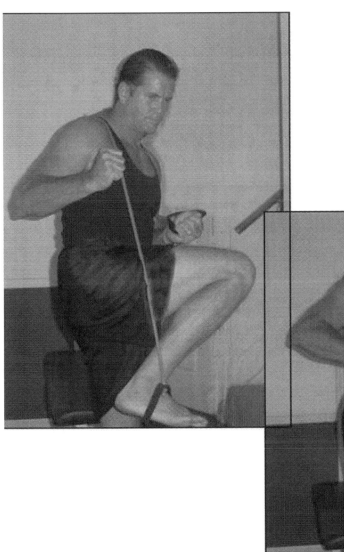

Here we practice a low side kick by wrapping the tube around the body, lifting the knee and then snapping it down. .

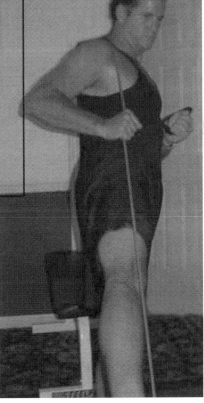

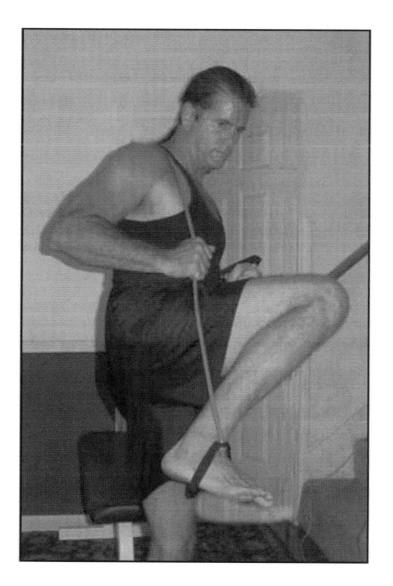

Here we practice a the side kicking posture. Holding the leg high and to the side. .

Here we practice a high round
kick, holding the wall for
support. . .

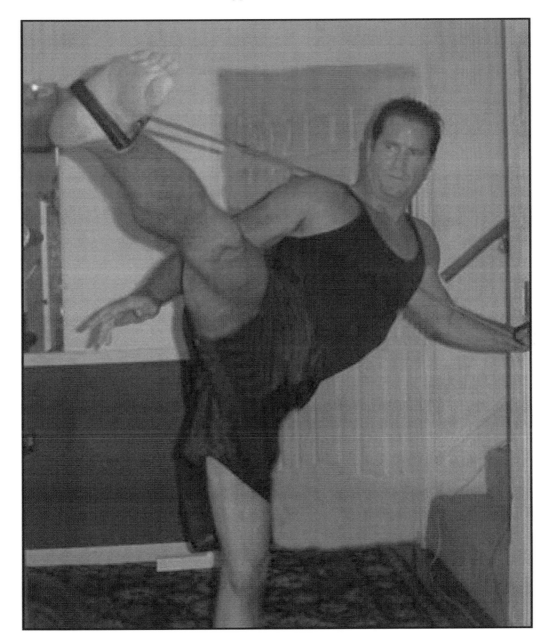

Here we practice a high round kick, holding the wall for support, be sure to hit with the heel or the ball of the foot.

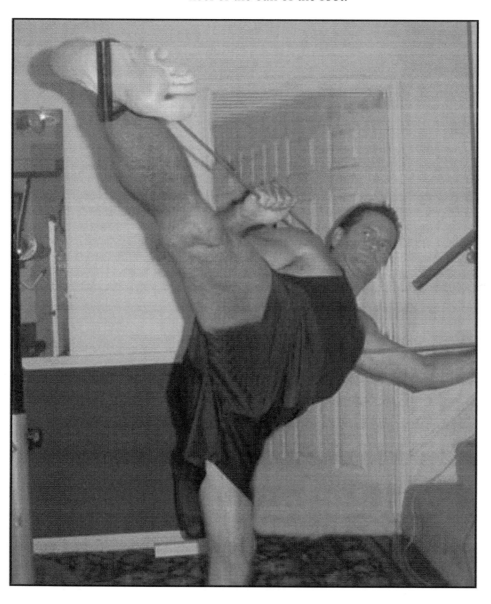

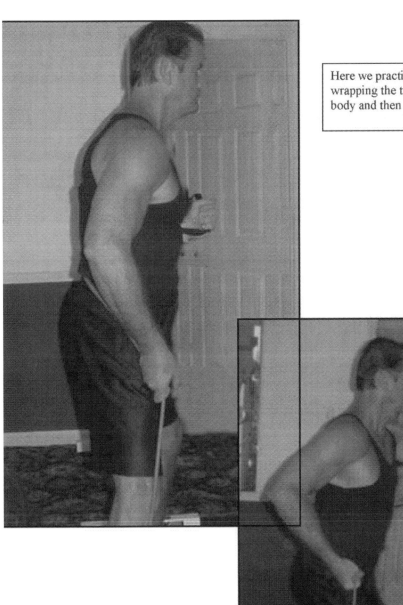

Here we practice a front punch, wrapping the tube around the body and then punching out.

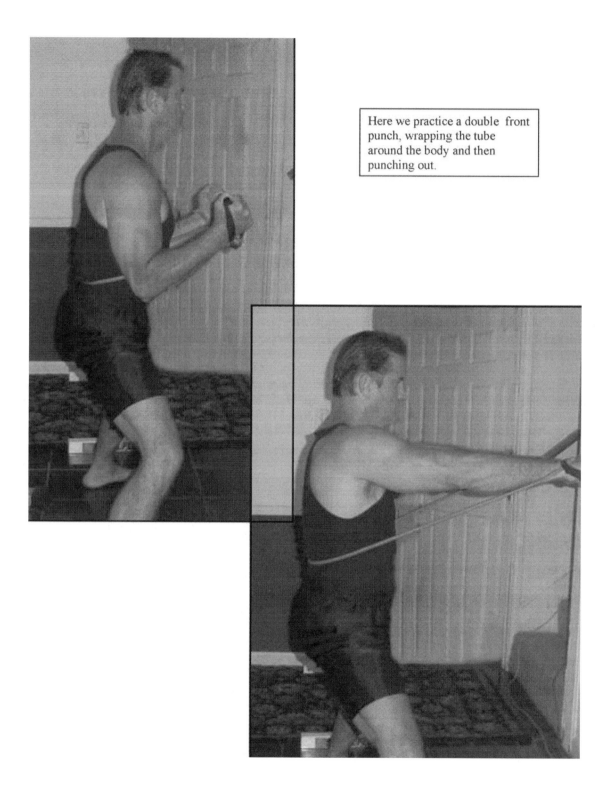

Here we practice a double front punch, wrapping the tube around the body and then punching out.

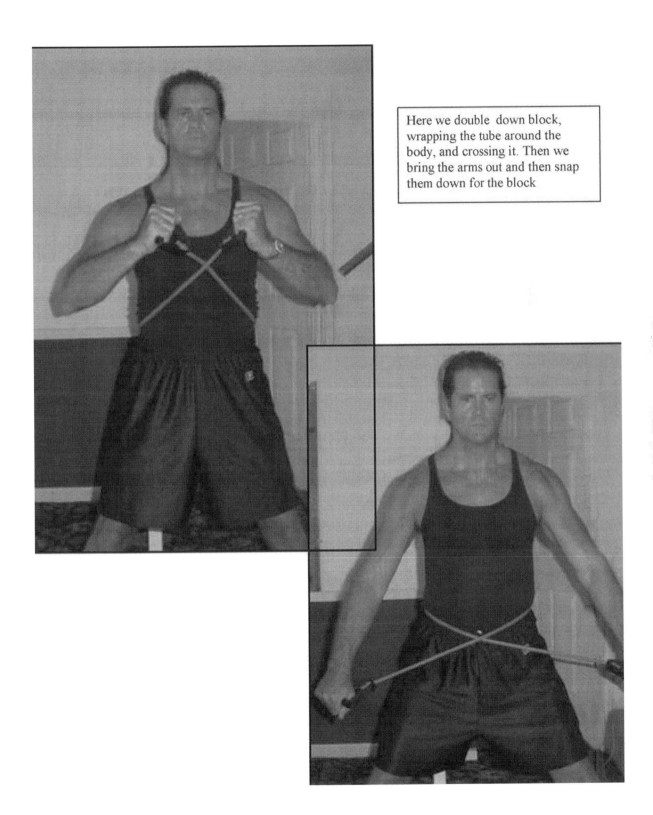

Here we double down block, wrapping the tube around the body, and crossing it. Then we bring the arms out and then snap them down for the block

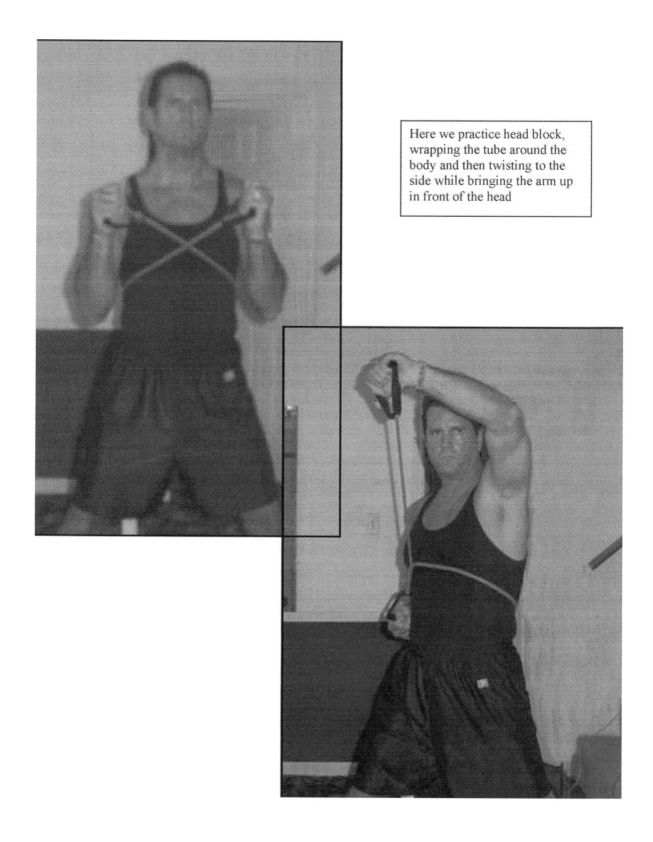

Here we practice head block, wrapping the tube around the body and then twisting to the side while bringing the arm up in front of the head

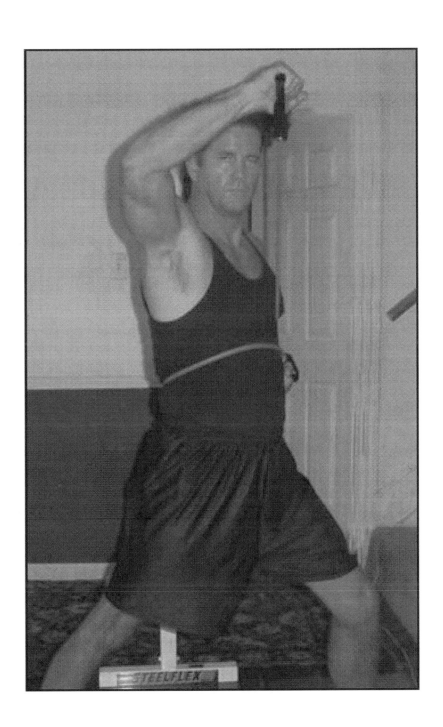

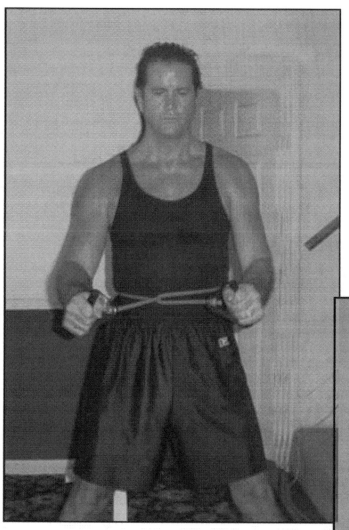

Here we practice side block wrapping the tube around the body and then twisting to the side while bringing the arm up and directly to the side, keeping the elbow in and pulling the other arm back.

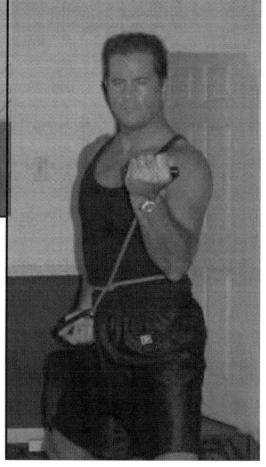

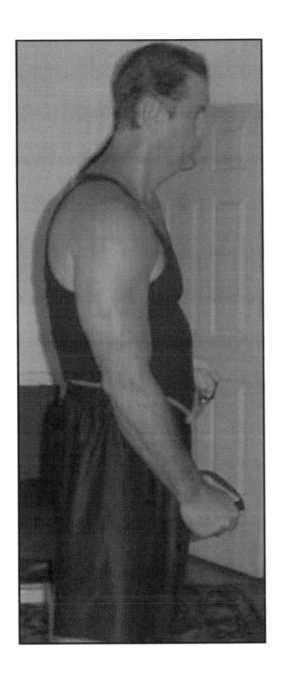

The side block shown from the side. Please notice the feet .

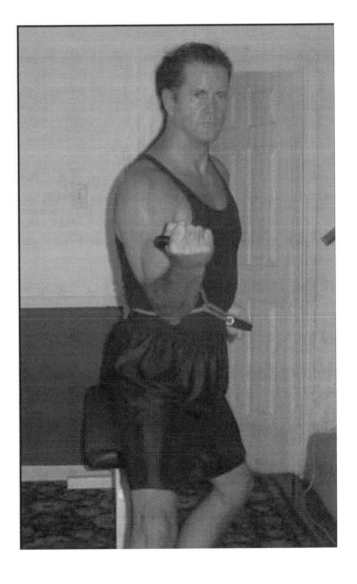

Here we practice the double down
block. Wrapping the tube around
the body and snapping the arms
down to the side.

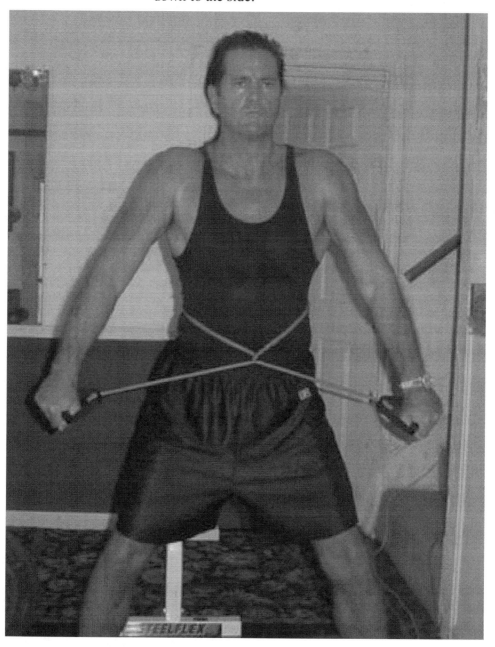

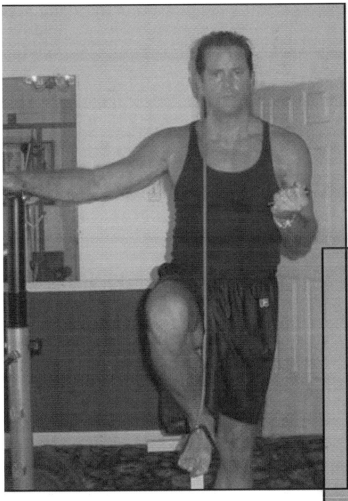

Here we practice a hard down leg snap kick. Holding the tube around the body, bringing the leg up and then snapping it down.

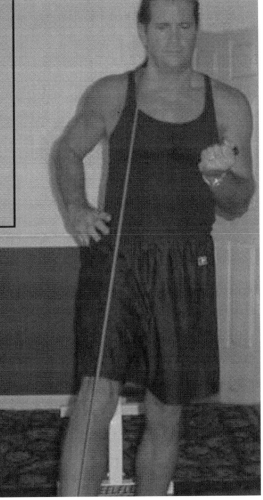

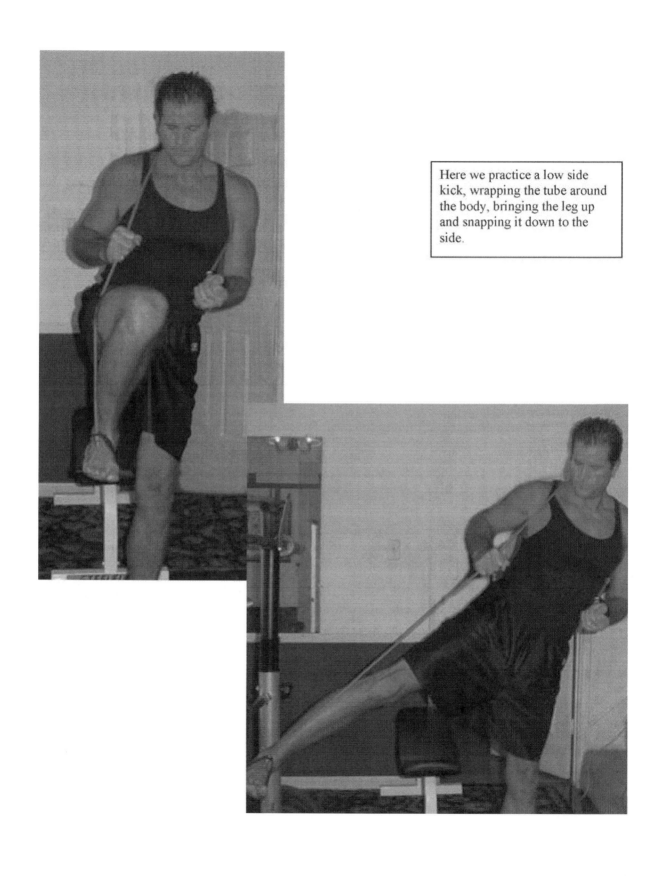

Here we practice a low side kick, wrapping the tube around the body, bringing the leg up and snapping it down to the side.

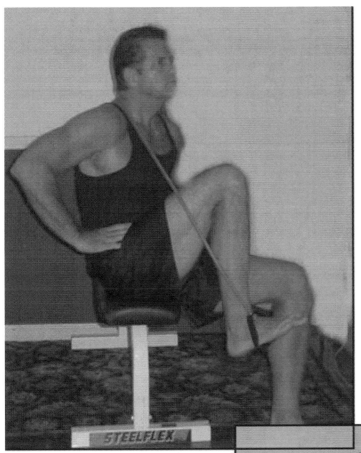

Here we practice sitting front snap, wrapping the tube around the body, bringing the leg up and snapping it out forward.

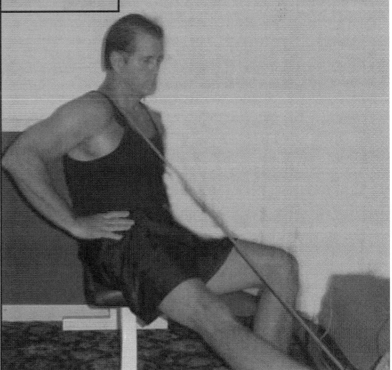

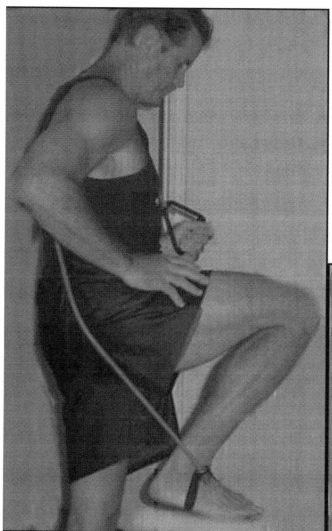

Here we practice low foot stomp. Lifting the leg high and then snapping it down

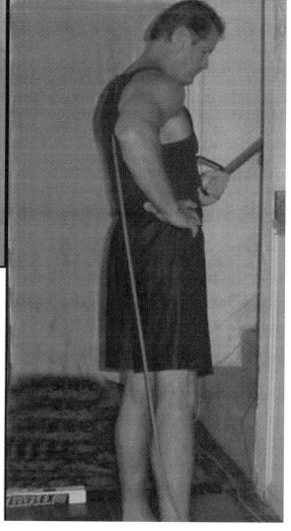

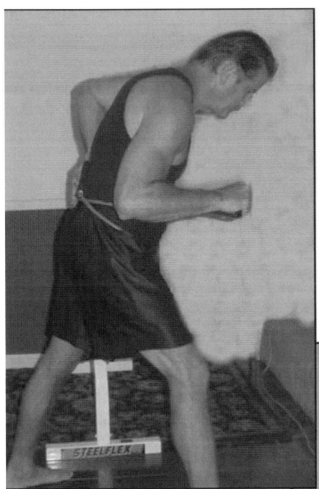

Here we a low punch, wrapping the tube around the body then leaning forward and thrusting the arm down and out.

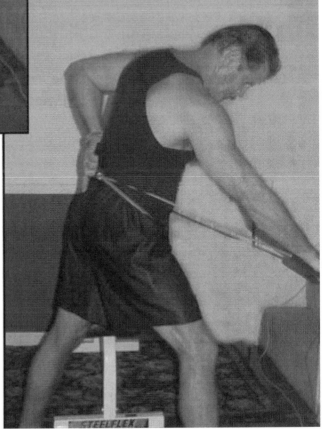

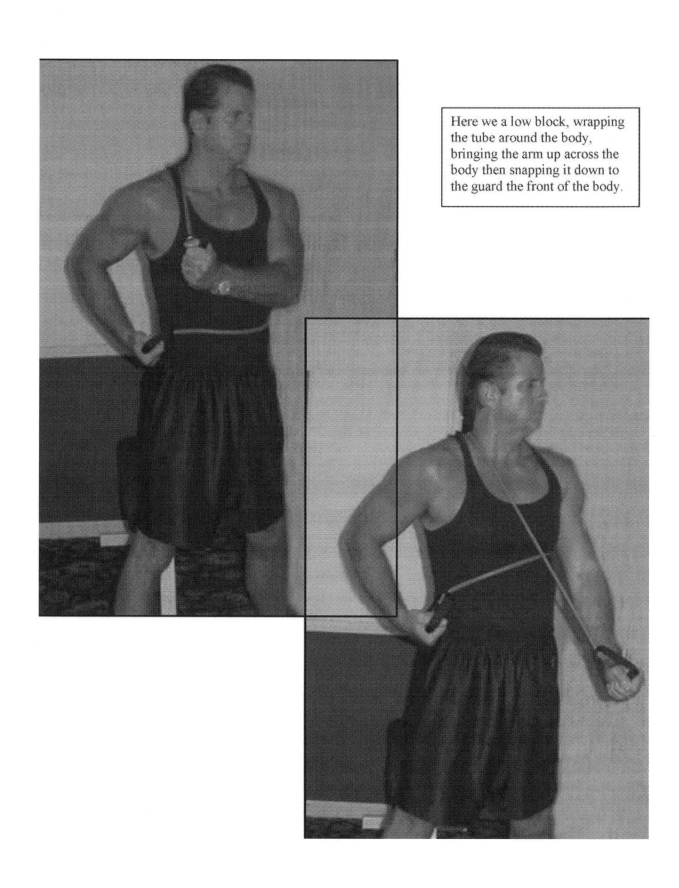

Here we a low block, wrapping the tube around the body, bringing the arm up across the body then snapping it down to the guard the front of the body.

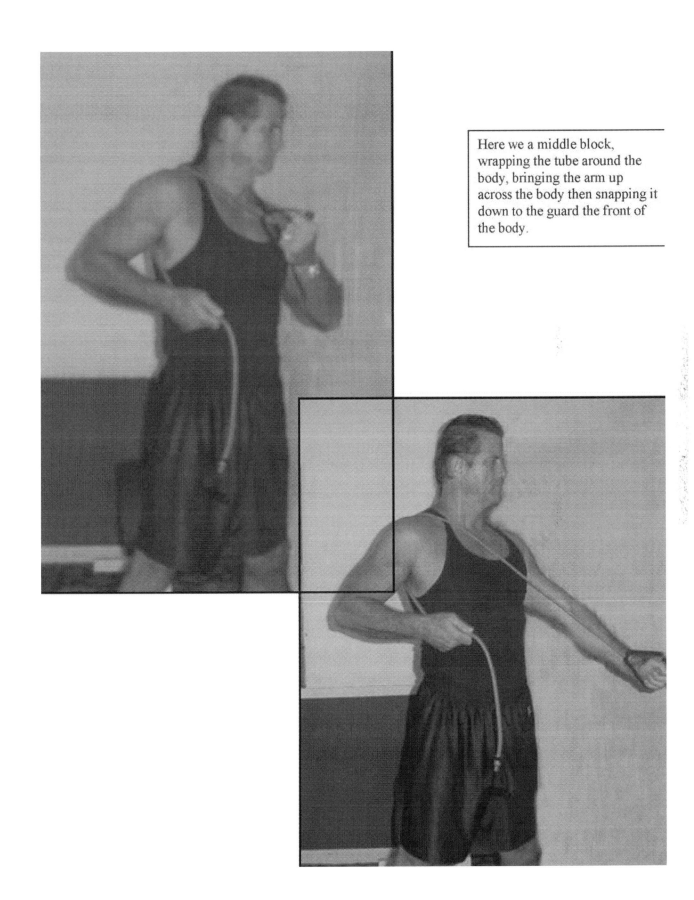

Here we a middle block, wrapping the tube around the body, bringing the arm up across the body then snapping it down to the guard the front of the body.

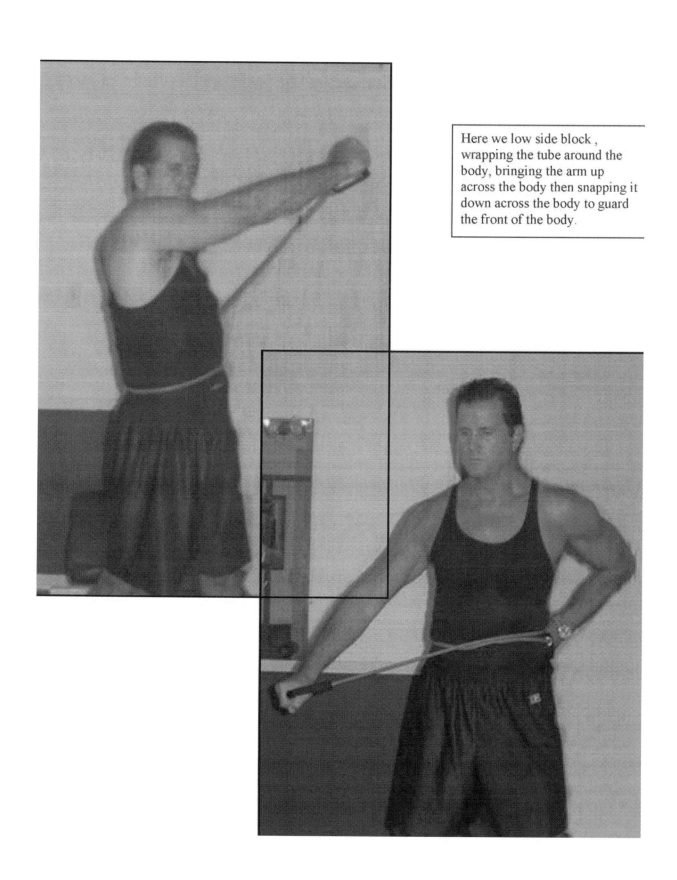

Here we low side block , wrapping the tube around the body, bringing the arm up across the body then snapping it down across the body to guard the front of the body.

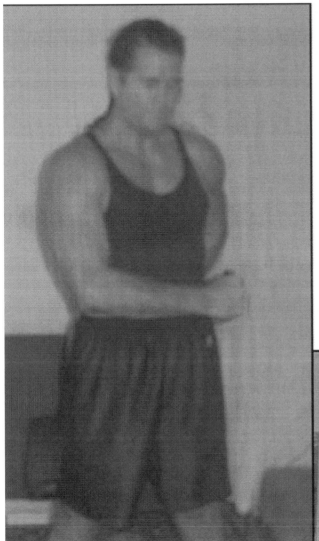

Here we middle block , wrapping the tube around the body, bringing the arm up across the body then snapping it down across the body to guard the front of the body.

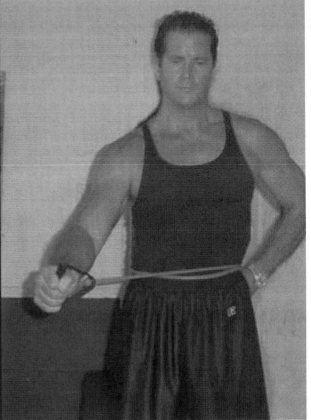

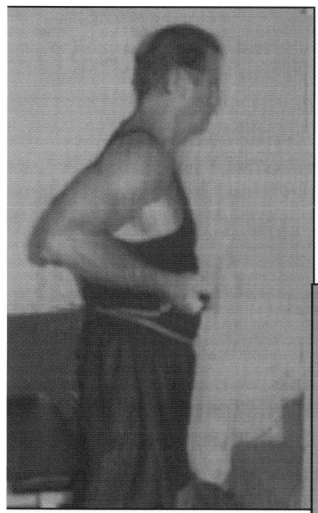

Here we middle upper punch. wrapping the tube around the body, holding the arm by the side and then snapping the arm up to the center of the body. .

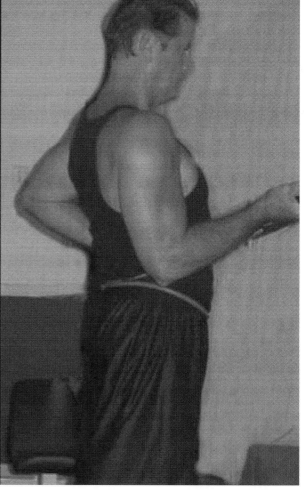

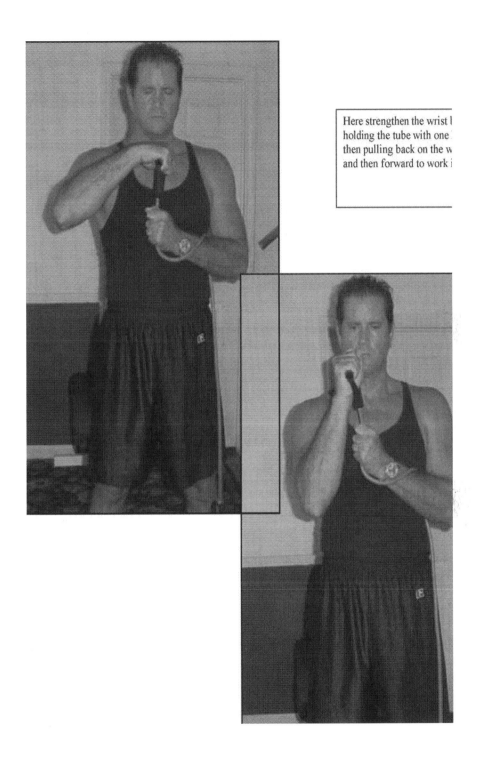

Here strengthen the wrist
holding the tube with one
then pulling back on the w
and then forward to work i

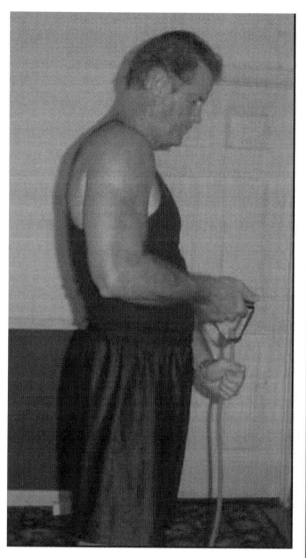

Here strengthen the wrist by holding the tube with one hand then pulling back on the wrist and then forward to work it. .

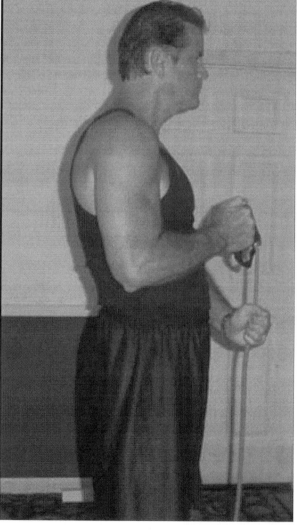

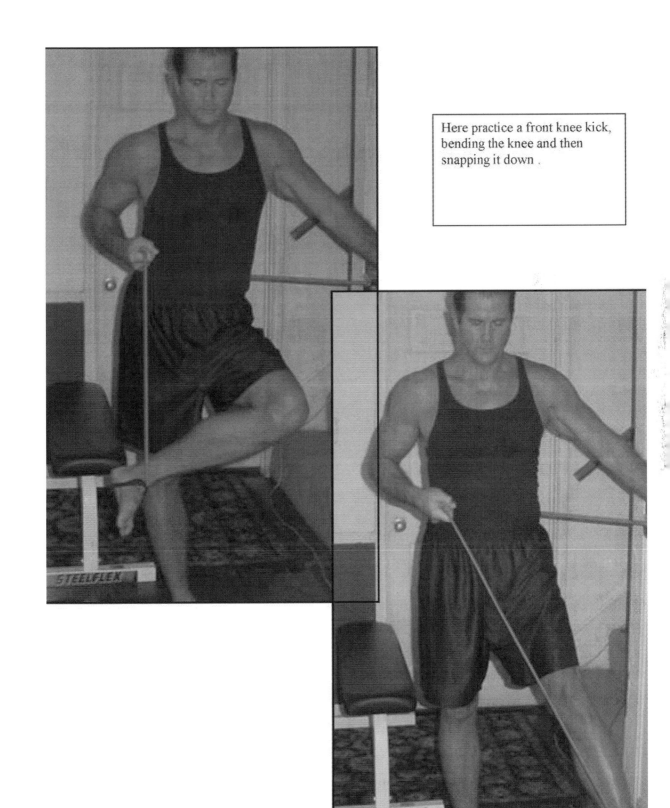

Here practice a front knee kick, bending the knee and then snapping it down .

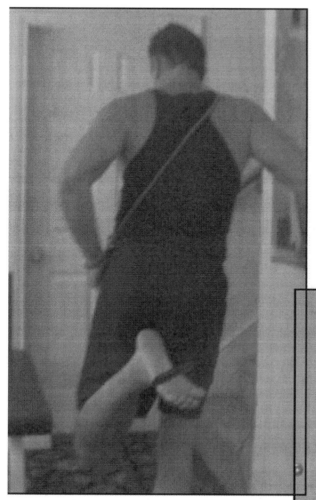

Here we practice a back kick, wrapping the tube around the foot and then leaning forward while kicking back.

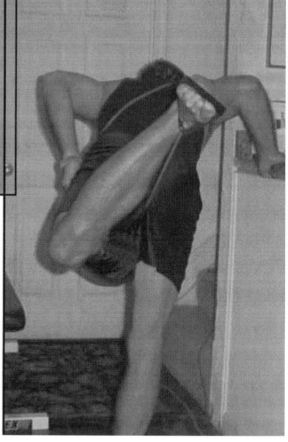

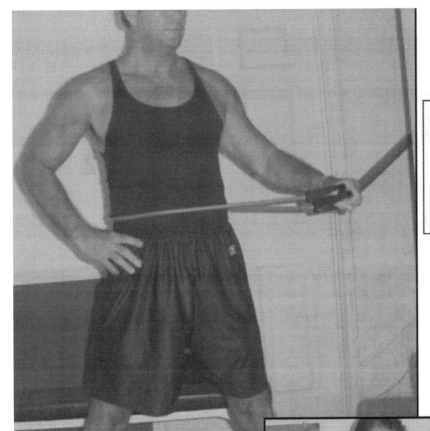

Here work our hip snap.
Holding the tube around the
body with one arm out, we twist
hard to the side and snap back
with the hips, this builds our hip
strength for punching and
kicking. .

Here work our hip snap.
Holding the tube around the
body with one arm out, we twist
hard to the side and snap back
with the hips, this builds our hip
strength for punching and
kicking. .

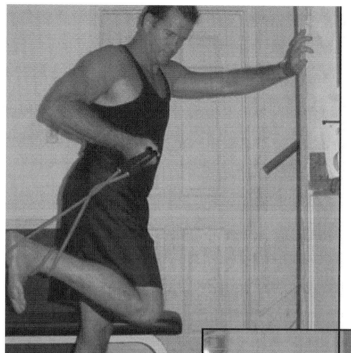

Here we practice our low snap, by holding the leg up and then snapping it down.

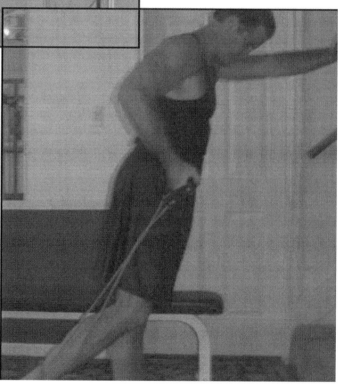

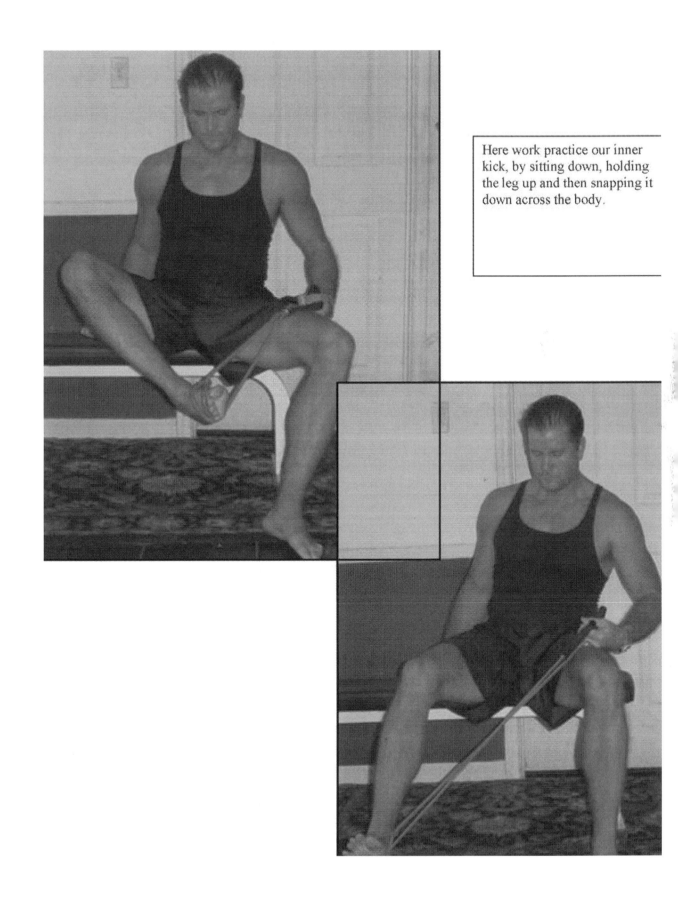

Here work practice our inner kick, by sitting down, holding the leg up and then snapping it down across the body.

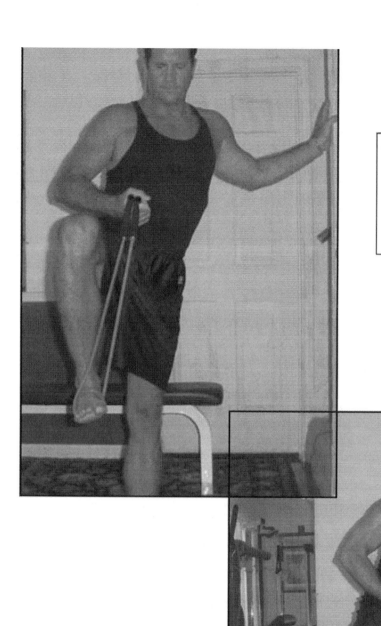

Here work our hip kick. Holding the leg up, we snap the foot backward to break the knee.

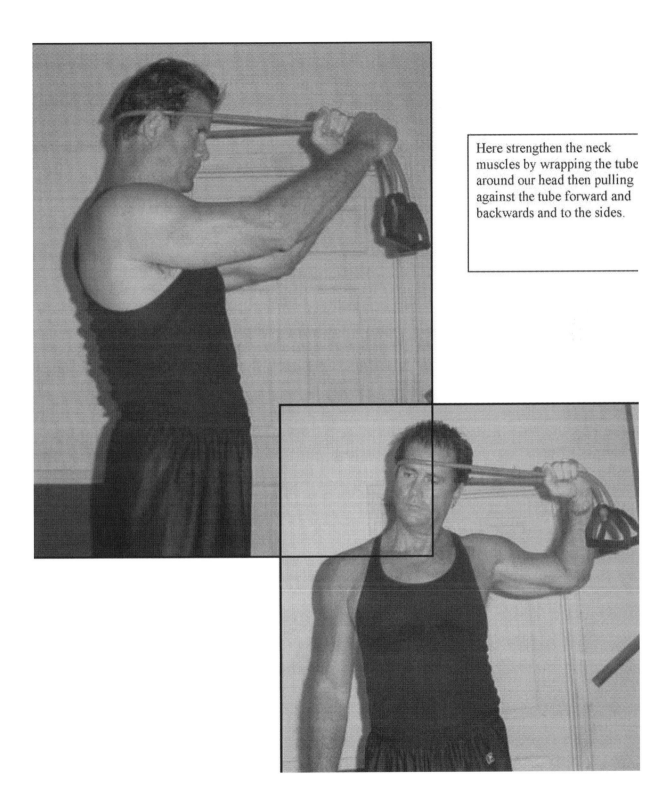

Here strengthen the neck muscles by wrapping the tube around our head then pulling against the tube forward and backwards and to the sides.